HOW NOT TO TEAR YOUR
FAMILY
APART

3 Simple Steps to Start Critical Conversations and
Help Your Family and Aging Parents Plan a
Financially Stable Future

Jason,

good Luck,

Carroll

CARROLL S. GOLDEN

Distribution by Bublish, Inc.

ISBN: 978-1-647044-24-4 (paperback)
ISBN: 978-1-647044-23-7 (eBook)

DEDICATION

This book is dedicated to my children, Erik and Nicole. My son and daughter never complain about the many hours that I spend working. Instead, they offer me constant support, love, and encouragement, and they help me believe that our tomorrows are filled with possibilities.

Heartfelt appreciation to my generational family: my sisters and their husbands for gracefully aging alongside me; my daughter-in-law Jodi; and Carolyn, James, Lyndsey, Norah, and Colton for their unreserved affection in teaching me about generations to come.

ACKNOWLEDGMENTS

Thanks to my many personal and professional friends for their influence, sharing of knowledge, and inspiration. I am grateful to the leadership and participants of the Long-term Care Insurance Section of the Society of Actuaries and the Intercompany Long-term Care Insurance Conference for the many years of contributing and fostering a continual expansion of long-term care knowledge, innovation, and education.

Thank you, Kevin Mayeux, CEO of the National Association of Insurance and Financial Advisors (NAIFA), for inspiring the creation of the Limited and Extended Care Planning (LECP) Center. Along with the team at NAIFA and sponsors of the LECP Center, the LECP Center strives to offer outstanding resources so advisors and consumers have access to actionable ideas and information.

I appreciate the collaboration and support offered by Sharon Reed, Steve Cain, Tom Reiske, David Kikoen, Nicole Stuart, Erik Deer, James Shea, Shelley Giordano, Dan Mangus, Betty Meredith, and Joe Dowdall. Thank you all for reviewing the book for readability and content.

Special thanks to Towera Loper for her kindness in sharing her wisdom, Suzanne Carawan for her inspiration and creativity, and Byron Holtz for his belief in my know-how.

Without the generous guidance of Kathy Meis, my publisher, there would not be a book to share. Although I published numerous articles, working with a first-time book author is not an easy task. Her continual encouragement, stress-free access to her expertise and guidance, her deep knowledge of the publishing industry, along with her patience and sense of humor, were essential to bringing my words to life.

DISCLAIMER

Neither the author nor the other contributors offer this information as tax, legal, investment, or retirement advice or recommendations. You are encouraged to seek guidance from an independent tax, investment, or legal professional. The content is derived from sources believed to be accurate. All links and references were in working order as of the publication date. Neither the information presented nor any opinion expressed constitutes a solicitation for the purchase or sale of any product or security. Interpretation of planning tools and products are used in the context of the family story but may be suitable for other planning situations as well. Please consult an investment advisor, tax consultant, or attorney before making a tax-related investment/insurance decision.

CONTENTS

SECTION III: A GROWING MARKETPLACE OFFERS EXPANDING OPTIONS AND PLANNING TOOLS

INTRODUCTION

My History

I have been an advisor in the life and health-care industry for many years. After seeing how a lack of planning can destroy even the most stable of families, I decided to specialize in long-term care. I discovered that individuals do not define "long-term " as an actual span of time but more by how well prepared the recipient and/or someone else is to recognize and manage care needs. Physical, emotional, and financial resources can quickly be exhausted. Stress can make a short amount of time feel like an eternity. I will use the terms *extended* or *long-term care* throughout this book because those terms accurately capture the reality of the need for multiple generations to plan for longer lives with growing psychological, financial, and health-care implications.

As a professional, I became more and more interested in long-term care because it mixes multigenerational emotions with multigenerational logic. Familiar with the psychological and emotional aspects from personal experience, I plunged into investing in my growth as a professional. Early in my career, I enrolled in courses at the highly respected American College of Financial Services. I earned the Chartered Life Underwriter® (CLU®) and the Chartered Financial Consultant® (ChFC®) designations, which incorporate information and practical applications in the form of case studies around tax, retirement, and investment strategies. To increase my long-term care knowledge, I earned the Certification in Long-Term Care® (CLTC®) designation, which includes education in the fields of insurance, financial services, law, and accounting. Another specialized course, offered by America's Health Insurance Plans (AHIP), earned me the Long-Term Care Professional® (LTCP®) designation. Seeking to broaden my grasp of issues related to the "graying of America," I returned to the American College of Financial Services, where I earned the Chartered Advisor in Senior Living® (CASL®) designation, which is committed to helping aging clients achieve financial security now and into the future. While holding leadership positions in both major insurance companies and distribution agencies specializing in long-term care, I earned the Fellow, Life Management Institute® (FLMI®) designation, which is a ten-course professional development program that provides an industry-specific business education in the context of the insurance and financial services industry. Recently, I received the Life and Annuity Certified Professional® (LACP®) designation from the National Association of Insurance and Financial Advisors (NAIFA), a certification that requires knowledge and experience beyond the requirements for industry licensure. Additionally, every two years, I complete my state's continuing education licensure requirements, affording me the opportunity to learn and interact directly with consumers and advisors/agents.

I also gain insights from teaching, working, and holding leadership positions in professional associations. As a member of the Society of Financial Service Professionals (FSP), I served as a chapter president and taught continuing education (CE) classes. I was the chairperson for the Society of Actuaries® (SOA) Fifth Long-Term Care Conference, and five years later, I chaired the Intercompany Long-term Care Insurance Conference (ILTCI). As a speaker for the Retirement Speakers Bureau[1] and for NAIFA's Limited and Extended Care Planning (LECP) Center, I enjoy offering interactive webinars on various extended and long-term care consumer planning options. I am responsible for creating and offering the Long-Term Care Insurance module for the Plan4Life/Salem University program, which leads to a professional certification as an Elder Planning Specialist. I serve as the Executive Director of NAIFA's LECP Center. Supporters of NAIFA and the LECP Center represent different points in the continuum of care, but they share a common purpose and mission to maximize professional and consumer awareness and the distribution of limited and extended care planning options at a time when it is a growing generational American need.

I have two very smart sisters who are not close in age. Creating plans for them and their families meant learning to work with two different generations, both of whom were already busy with family, volunteer work, careers, and friends. It required me to broaden my familiarity with established and newer care options and to hone my ability to work with different budgets and different lifestyles.

My son and daughter reminded me about the shoemaker who had no shoes. I needed to plan for myself. I found myself working with yet another generation, viewing life through their younger, simpler lens. It was and continues to be my most valuable lesson. From them, I learned the value of clear communication. Different generations attach different meanings to words and phrases, learning words and expressions in the context of their experience, which may or may not be a shared experience.

My family's extended and long-term care planning provided me with hands-on experience—and, just as significantly, so did the family situation into which I remarried. I know what you are thinking: "You are so knowledgeable in this area that it must have been easy for you." As you will see, it was informative but not easy. Additional lessons and insights were on the horizon. My in-laws had a history of both Alzheimer's disease and longevity in their gene pools. While advances in medicine and science have had a positive effect on longevity, diseases of the brain, unfortunately, have seen only marginal improvements. My husband's father suffered from Alzheimer's disease. Alzheimer's disease is the most common form of dementia. It causes problems with memory, thinking, and behavior. There are three progressive stages:

mild, moderate, and severe. To varying degrees, he lost his ability to respond to his environment, remain in control of his movements, or carry on a conversation. The gene for Alzheimer's disease can be inherited. This scary thought exacerbated the difficulty of planning for aging and made family conversations uncomfortable. Unspoken issues can be a communication stopper. We had to focus on options, not on the possibility of the disease being passed on. On the other hand, my mother-in-law came from a family with a history of longevity, with relatives living well into their late nineties.

What is true for so many families was true for them. As a newcomer to the family, I surmised that there were several challenges to moving ahead with planning. No one was comfortable starting the conversation about these important topics. No one knew what to say or how to engage in an open dialogue. No one wanted to make our family's maturing members feel bad because of their potential care needs or feel like they were being punished for living a long life. No one wanted them to feel like they were being "managed" or "handled." Maybe no one felt like they had the know-how to even find a suitable advisor or specialist. Maybe they googled long-term care and became overwhelmed by everything that needed to be considered. No matter what caused the hesitation, it had a huge and very negative impact on my new family's finances and emotional cohesiveness. Discourse and disagreements about planning led to no planning. Later, when my mother-in-law needed care, the family could not agree on anything. The smallest decision led to awkward silences or nasty commentary.

I experienced firsthand how the lack of communication about family generational planning is exhausting, painful, and sad. I discovered many families think that planning for care is unaffordable or would involve a long, drawn-out process.

My Objective

A major objective of my three simple steps is to avoid counterproductive family stress or conflict while trying to create an actionable plan. If you don't know your options, you cannot see how to move forward. I'll provide an overview to broaden your familiarity with several currently available options that could fit almost any budget.

The industry's use of insurance lingo may cause you to back off a conversation. I have tried to explain insurance and government program lingo in simple terms, but a deep dive with a professional is advised.

Families already come loaded with lots of built-in dynamics. We all know that too many players on a playing field can create confusion. My three simple steps create a game plan. All players are invited to the game, and everyone knows their role. Individual aptitudes, lifestyle demands, and availability are acknowledged. Just like a successful team, everyone in the family (however you define family) knows their role and respects others. In the end, what will you have to show for engaging in my simple, three-step process?

- You avoid singling out any family member or generation as "needy."
- Your family uses this book to start the conversation about planning for the future.
- You use an inclusive rather than an exclusive approach, which means everyone feels good about, or at least accepts, the plan because they were part of the process.
- You establish leadership and rules so things can move forward.
- You identify the best available options.
- The financial burden doesn't fall on any one family member or friend.
- You are prepared if sudden or longer term care is needed.

- No family member or friend feels guilty because they can't interrupt their lives or live too far away to provide care.
- You become an educated consumer and consult a professional when you need more in-depth information or advice.

During the COVID-19 pandemic, we saw two realities confirmed. First, no one is immune to sudden, unexpected care events. Second, most of us are unprepared for limited, extended, or long-term illness care needs. We all know that preparation is key and could have helped many families cope more effectively with some of the situations that COVID-19 presented or in which they find themselves as their parents age.

The goal of this book is to help individuals, families, and friends plan for both the expected and unexpected. Use this book as a tool to broaden your understanding of how to start important conversations with friends and family about long-term planning and to learn about your options. In the case of planning for immediate, extended, or long-term care needs, one size does *not* fit all. To bring to life the gravity of some of the issues facing families as they undertake this planning, I've created the Jones family, whose stories will hopefully demonstrate how all this works in the real world. There are three generations in the Jones family: the grandparents, James and Carolyn; their daughter and son-in-law, Jodi and Jackson; and their grandchildren, Erik and Nicole. I hope you'll see yourself or someone you care about in some of these characters and be inspired to share this book with others who need to start important generational conversations and open a planning dialogue with friends and/or family.

My three simple steps offer you a framework to start conversations, open lines of communication, encourage participation, and talk about choices and financial stability. This is about living your best possible life as you age and letting other generations do the same.

SECTION

I

Overview

CHAPTER 1

The Earlier You Plan, the More Options You Have

Currently, many families both in the United States and abroad are caring for a parent while also caring for immediate family members and the generation beneath them. It's a natural life cycle. The term *sandwich generation* has been around for a long time, but comprehending its meaning is more important than ever with science and medical advances keeping us alive longer. This has put more adults with children *and* aging parents or close friends in the middle of a complicated juggling act.

Longevity is a blessing that exacerbates and intensifies the need to plan for extended or long-term care—and we're not just talking about health-care needs. There are also lifestyle needs. The need to age in a setting that allows for interaction with others to avoid depression or misplaced anger is well documented. Loneliness and isolation can be deadly, literally. There are also financial needs. Worrying about running out of money or being forced to move out of familiar surroundings is stressful. These issues ripple through a family's financial stability and relationships. From a macroeconomic and cultural viewpoint, these shifts are impacting societal norms. According to the Pareto principle, 80 percent of the consequences stem from 20 percent of the causes. One family member, or one close friend, who looks to you for help with extended or long-term care needs can impact your life in ways you don't anticipate. The COVID-19 pandemic was a nasty wake-up call for the entire world. It opened all of our eyes to the limitations of the government, the health-care system, and even families' abilities to provide safe and adequate care when things go wrong at a local, state, national, or global level.

The earlier you plan, the more options you have. Some options may not be available if you wait to plan and most certainly will be more expensive. Various options are linked to your chronological age. If you plan early, you may have time to amass needed funds for an option that suits you. Planning early helps you understand how government programs may be integrated into a plan. Some options depend on your good health. It is usually easier to qualify at younger ages. Still other options are available to you as a homeowner if you plan to age at home. Planning early may allow you to move taxable savings into a long-term care program, which may ameliorate the tax hit. The sooner the better is the best timing for extended and long-term care planning.

Takeaway:

However you define family, unplanned extended and long-term care issues ripple and/or rip through a family's financial stability and relationships. The only remedy is to plan; and the best plan is a result of becoming organized and educated about which options work best for your situation.

CHAPTER 2

Finding Your Motivation to Plan

When you're reading the Jones family's stories, you might be reminded of your own family or friends. Members of the Jones family have noticed that the grandparents are showing signs of aging, but they aren't sure how to start the difficult conversation they need to have about planning for the future. The family uses the three steps outlined in this book to have "the talk" and navigate their options. The generations in this family are forced to pull together despite their differences. Attitudes, beliefs, habits, experiences, values, and especially communication and comprehension differ from one generation to the next. The steps in this book help them learn to solve issues together and build relationships based on learning to hear and understand one another. The goal is to effectively plan the best care outcome for their loved ones. This means they must work together as a team to address the many safety, health-care, financial, and lifestyle decisions ahead.

Is starting this important family conversation easy? No, it is not. It's awkward and difficult, but it is absolutely necessary. Everyone needs to have this dialogue—and do so as soon as possible. There are literally thousands, if not millions, of reports, disturbing statistics, and heartbreaking tales of financial ruin, generational infighting, and caregiver burnout. Unfortunately, the odds are stacked against you and time is not on your side. For most families, it takes a scary, sad, or upsetting experience to push everyone into action. By then, unfortunately, it's often too late to avoid some of the worst consequences of the family's delayed action. That's why it is so important to stay ahead of the curve. Without a plan, your family risks the following:

- Negative impacts on family members' lifestyles. What if a parent must move in with you or if you must move in with a parent in need of care?
- Diminished Social Security benefits and investment savings as the family caregiver devotes time to caregiving instead of earning income.
- Depletion of retirement savings.
- Delays in education funding for younger generations.
- On-the-job stress or employment absences due to caregiving requirements and emergencies.
- Decreased cash flow, leading to limited care options.
- Diminished assets values resulting from a fire sale situation.
- Compelled asset liquidation when the market timing isn't good, resulting in unwanted taxation.
- Limited potential future investment growth due to diminished invested funds.
- Retirees and pre-retirees unable to preserve the money they have worked so hard to save for their legacy.
- Feeling guilty because you didn't have the conversation with your parents or spouse, and their choices are now less attractive or not possible because of poor or no planning.

You want a funded plan in place as early as possible so that you are in control of the type of care, the care setting, and the care services you want for your future self or the older members of your family. You also want these choices without breaking the bank. The earlier your family plans together, the more likely it is that you will avoid painful outcomes as your family ages.

This book offers a generational primer to save families the heartache, financial shock, stress, discord, and ongoing conflict that the absence of long-term planning often causes.

For many people, planning for extended or long-term care lacks a driving force until it's too late. In addition to the motivators listed, the COVID-19 pandemic and images of the shortages of health and wellness services were a wake-up call for many of us. If these realities aren't a trigger for you, then let me be clear: You need to have these important family conversations today and move toward a plan as soon as possible.

Takeaway:

It's really never too early to start planning, but it's frequently too late. Use this book as a tool and commit to starting these crucial conversations today instead of tearing your family apart.

CHAPTER 3

How to Use This Book

G iven the different stages of planning and different generational compositions of each family, you will want to individualize the information and guidance in this book. However, these three simple steps—the book's foundation—can be used in any order. We will follow the Jones family as they personalize the steps, resources, and tools to create a plan that fits their family's needs, budget, and goals. Here are the three steps to get started.

Step One: Create a Care Guide

Plan for immediate family care needs by creating a Care Guide filled with current, accurate information about each member of your family. It's a great place to start for yourself, your children, and your aging parents. The guide can be handed to doctors, health-care workers, and other service professionals in times of urgent need. Care Guides eliminate stress by consolidating and organizing crucial, up-to-date information. Creating a Care Guide is also a great way to get everyone working together and start those difficult conversations regarding health and safety. It's the "*I care*" conversation. Someone may not remember what you said, but they will remember how you made them feel. The process of creating family Care Guides is the perfect icebreaker to kickstart planning.

Step Two: Select a Care Squad

The objective of the Care Squad is to create a process for family members to react effectively when emergencies arise. It's the "*what if*" conversation. A Care Squad can help families avoid chaos and delays in a crisis situation. The Care Squad designates who does what when something goes wrong. Who goes over to Mom and Dad's house to be with them? Who calls the doctor or an ambulance? Who's in charge of handing over the Care Guide to health-care professionals? Who contacts other family members or friends? You get the idea. Everyone knows their role in advance and can spring into action with a clear understanding of how they can help.

Step Three: Assign a Care Planning Team

> "Fight for the things that you care about, but do it
> in a way that will lead others to join you."
> —Ruth Bader Ginsberg

The Care Planning Team (CPT) provides a multigenerational structure for discussion and assessment in the long-term care planning process. CPT members each have a voice. As a group, they research available options that suit each generation's immediate, extended, or long-term care needs. The generational diversity of the group encourages and requires respect and an understanding of different lifestyles and generational priorities. It's the *"discovery"* conversation. When it is time to seek professional advice or support, the CPT members should be educated consumers—ready to discuss options, ask relevant questions, and make decisions.

These three simple steps are achievable. They provide a gateway to important conversations that are often hard to start but are always better to have before a crisis hits. Even though the Jones family is fictitious, these scenarios play out every day. Hopefully, seeing the Jones family work through their issues, choices, and roadblocks will inspire you and give you courage to take the first step in the planning process with multigenerational family members and/or friends.

Takeaway:

My mission is to demystify the extended and long-term care planning process and to provide actionable information that you can use to help your family prepare for a financially stable future. The emphasis is on uncovering potential options and not on recommending specific financial products or services. Products and services may apply differently to your situation and new products and services will be introduced over time, but my hope is this story increases your familiarity with available options and moves you to action. Knowledge is a powerful tool.

SECTION

II

Plan. Don't Panic!

CHAPTER 4

Meet James and Carolyn Jones

Traditionally, retirement meant leaving a 9-to-5 job and living out your golden years. Social security income and pensions supported the retiree's lifestyle. People retired from their job but did not retire from their family.

Life expectancy throughout most of human evolution was somewhere between eighteen and twenty years. Life was short. By the mid-1800s life expectancy had reached the mid-thirties in the United States, and in 1900 it was forty-seven years. By the end of the twentieth century, life expectancy had reached seventy-seven years. It gained thirty years in one century—that's unprecedented.[2] The increase in life expectancy made family caregiving for elderly people more common.

Being a part of the silent generation has shaped the value system and lifestyle predilections of Grandpa James and Grandma Carolyn. Born between 1928 and 1945, the silent generation were children of the Great Depression whose parents, having reveled in the highs of the Roaring Twenties, faced great economic hardship and struggled to provide for their families. Silents, as the people of this generation were called, grew up seeing the ravages of war and plummeting financial markets. This led them to develop a strong will to work hard and save money. Unlike the previous generation, who had fought to change the system, the silent generation worked within the system. They kept their heads down and worked hard, thus earning themselves the "silent" label. Their attitudes leaned toward not being risk-takers and playing it safe.[3] This attitude influences conversations and ideas from the outset.

Our modern-day concept of retirement developed due to a combination of increased life spans, advances in medicine and the treatment of diseases, the growing popularity of pension plans in certain sectors, and the onset of government-sponsored benefits in 1935 with the creation of Social Security.[4] Typical of the silent generation, Grandpa James and Grandma Carolyn expect social security income and company pensions to be a major source of retirement income. Many silents also assume their children will be their caregivers. As a result, rooms for grandparents and in-law suites had become more common.

A new demographic of family caregiver is emerging, and it may not be what you think it is. Lynn Feinberg, AARP senior strategic advisor, said, "Caregiving [is] not just a woman's issue: 40% of caregivers are men, 40% represent multicultural diversity and more millennials are taking on these tasks as well."[5] Older adults are also key providers of family care.[6] Grandpa James takes care of Grandma Carolyn, at least for now.

Today's generations are increasingly mobile. If you live an hour or more away from a person who needs care, consider yourself a long-distance caregiver. How will you identify and evaluate community and local agency resources? As care needs become more evident, you may feel guilty about not being available. If you have the burden of travel added to the other burdens of caregiving, will you become even less available to children, other family members, friends, and coworkers?

"Many long-distance caregivers act as information coordinators, helping aging parents understand the confusing maze of new needs, including home health aides, insurance benefits and claims, and durable medical equipment. Caregiving, no matter where the caregiver lives, is often long-lasting and ever-expanding. For the long-distance caregiver, what may start out as an occasional phone call to share family news can eventually turn into regular phone calls about managing household bills, getting medical information, and arranging for grocery deliveries. What begins as a monthly trip to check on Mom may become a larger project to move her to a new home or nursing facility closer to where you live."[7] As we will see, like the grandparent's daughter Jodi, many caregivers do not acknowledge the increasing burden of their caregiving duties. Others may not recognize the family's immediate, extended, and long-term care needs.

Grandma Carolyn and Grandpa Jones are retired. We haven't developed a word to describe the stage when retirement years morph into aging, when family and good friends slowly become dependent and need support. Following the three simple steps is a planning tool to encourage discussing and planning for pre-retirement and for all stages of retirement as well.

Takeaway:

Without a plan you may become the presumptive generational caregiver. The first frank conversation you need to have is with yourself. What can you do, and what can you not do?

CHAPTER 5

Recognizing Your Family's Immediate, Extended, and Long-Term Care Needs

As we move through life stages, family members (however you define family) take care of one another. It's what family is all about. Over the years and through the decades, we accept, prepare, and plan for the next step. Finally, we retire.

Nowadays, the term *retirement* can refer to a period that may stretch out twenty or thirty years. We generally accept that there are three common phases to retirement. How quickly you pass thorough the stages is influenced by your resources and health. In phase one, you may travel or pursue other activities that you put off due to family and career responsibilities. You may seek activities that add meaning or routine to life. The next phase may involve finding a community or living style that is more routine or settled. The third phase sees the effect of aging, but we still call it retirement. We lack a phrase to describe the stage when retirement years morph into aging, interdependency, and require increasing levels of assistance. Logically, retirement preparation should include preparing for long-term care needs. But few people prepare. Somehow this topic throws us for a loop. Why is preparing for this phase of life so daunting and intimidating?

Commonly, we fail to plan for the inevitable: Mom and Dad will age, probably live much longer than their parents did, and will likely require more specialized care over a longer period of time. Unfortunately, for many families, this combination has caused a perfect storm, pushing families' budgets and stress levels to the limit. More family caregivers are in the workforce—some 60 percent work full- or part-time in addition to their caregiving responsibilities. This trend will continue, and those who have to pull back face substantial economic risk from loss of income, benefits, contributions to their own retirement savings, or reduced social security benefits.[8]

Still, most people don't have a plan to deal with what's around the corner much less ten to fifteen years down the road. But then something happens. A father or grandparent becomes ill or can no longer live independently. A mother loses her job because she has had to take too much time off work to assist her aging parents. Something big happens and it's a wake-up call. If you're lucky, that wake-up call comes while there is still time to plan. If you're not so lucky, some profound changes are on the horizon and you're not well prepared to face them. It's this latter scenario that adds to the growing collection of nightmare stories that make their way into news headlines.

Let's check in on the Jones family to see how they handle some changes they're seeing.

> *Due to the pandemic, the Jones family canceled their annual barbecue. Unable to get together for a long time, they decide to celebrate Grandma Carolyn's seventy-seventh birthday on Zoom. At least a virtual party would be better than nothing.*

Generations

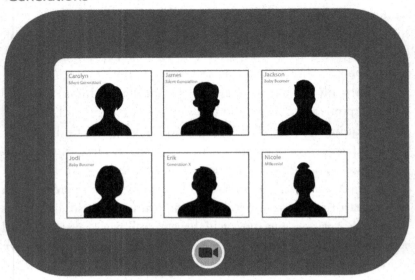

The entire four generations of the Jones family attend. Everyone enjoys the party, but they also notice Grandma Carolyn's frailty. Grandpa James had to help her stand up to blow out the candles on her birthday cake. Everything seemed to be moving in slow motion and everyone left the Zoom call concerned about Grandma Carolyn.

Grandma Carolyn's daughter, Jodi, is especially dismayed by what she saw. Over the last year, she has gradually taken on more and more caregiver duties, such as shopping, preparing meals, driving them to appointments that involve heavily trafficked or high-speed roads, speaking with doctors about treatments, running errands, doing laundry, and changing bed linens. It's been a gradual process. As a result, she doesn't really even associate all that she is doing with caregiving. Her father, James, always offers to help, but with his pacemaker and family history of heart failure, Jodi typically politely refuses.

Jodi's husband and two children see how each new responsibility takes its toll on Jodi. Sleep deprivation, unhealthy eating habits, and lack of exercise are just a few of the signs of her stress and overburdened schedule. After the birthday party, they fear that things are getting worse. Jodi's daughter, Nicole, even suspects that there also has been financial effects that her mom hasn't mentioned. She and her brother, Erik, talk and decide to take action before things get worse. Erik texts his sister a link to an article to use as a jumping off point for a conversation about planning for long-term care. They call their dad, Jackson, for advice. He explains that the topic is sort of taboo, but he offers to approach Jodi to start a conversation.

Grandma Carolyn, Grandpa James, and Jodi, two generations, are lucky that Erik and Nicole, the third generation, have the wherewithal to kickstart this important family conversation.

It's a typical situation. The grandparents have no plan in place, at least not one that the family knows about. What often happens without a plan is the care is self-funded by the senior and/or their spouse or partner until most or all assets are depleted. At that time, the person needing care may qualify for Medicaid, which is far from an optimal solution, or family members must start to dip into their own funds to pay for needed care. Sixty-eight percent of family caregivers have provided financial support, 93 percent have provided emotional support, and 90 percent have provided personal care support, such as hygiene and chores.[9] Knowing how to finance long-term care is essential, but it is obviously not the only issue.

A combination of demographic and economic shifts is creating a large and growing need for affordable and age-appropriate housing opportunities.

Most seniors would prefer not to leave familiar surroundings. Aging in place is another discussion best included early in planning. It's where most of us want to be—at home. Consider if the home might require a variety of costly and disruptive renovations. There is the issue of upkeep and social environment to consider, all of which can be decided and researched once critical conversations get started. It's so important to educate yourself about your options and to understand what this type of care setting involves.

More than 25 percent of seniors who need long-term care are not capable of making their own decisions when the time comes. Making those decisions for someone you love or are responsible for is an emotional burden that family members find extremely difficult. The impact of those decisions can linger for many years and often leads to family conflict.

What about being the caregiver? It is probably not a role for which you are trained. Forty-nine percent of caregivers experience feelings of depression. Fifty-seven percent of caregivers find it difficult to sleep on a regular basis.[10] Forty-six percent of caregivers have gained or lost weight as a result of caring for others.[11]

Do you think it won't happen to you or someone you love? Chances are you or someone in your family will need some level of extended or long-term care.[12] It's possible that 70 percent of us will need long-term care at some point.[13]

If you do not move forward with planning, many of the difficult, long-lasting consequences of not planning will become a part of your family's history. I see how confident my sisters, brothers-in-law, and our children are that our immediate family will be cared for without unduly burdening family members.

It's a conversation about how to help, instead of how to handle. It is hard to see a loved one lose their vitality, but it is unbearable to know you could have made the aging and care process more comfortable by planning and didn't get to it! Much is written about the first phase of retirement. Some even plan for the second phase, but it seems few of us want to acknowledge that the third phase requires advanced planning as well.

Takeaway:

If the topic of aging and care needs is taboo in your family or circle of friends, it is time to start talking. Use statistics, stories, or social media accounts to kick off the topic. Use the three simple steps to get organized and work on a real plan.

CHAPTER 6

Treading Lightly and Acknowledging the Need for Generational Planning

When it comes to extended and long-term care planning, starting the conversation is half the battle, as we see next with the Jones family.

Due to COVID-19 restrictions, the Jones family has not seen the cumulative effect that aging is having on Grandma Carolyn. The Zoom call shook everyone up. Everyone now realizes that a conversation is needed, except maybe Jodi, who is the caregiver. Caregivers often don't seek help until they become overwhelmed.

Jackson and Jodi sit down at the kitchen table to discuss if they should involve their entire family in the long-term care planning process.

"I know the kids want to help," Jodi explains, "but I can handle it."

"Jodi, I understand you want to shelter them, but they are family. They want to help. I'm not sure excluding them is the best course of action. I was reading about this in the news the other day. We're typical of the sandwich generation, supporting three generations at the same time—your parents, ourselves, and our children. You know how financially savvy our daughter, Nicole, is. Well, she sent me an article about the impact all of this could have on our retirement. It wasn't pretty, and she hesitated sending it to you."

"Why?" Jodi looks inquisitively at her husband.

"She doesn't want to upset you. She doesn't want you to think she's meddling," Jackson responds, placing his hand on his wife's arm. "Jodi, this is impacting everyone. Not saying anything to our children just makes them worry even more."

"OK," Jodi stiffens while trying not to sound defensive. "Please show me what she sent."

Jackson nudges the article toward his wife.

Top Financial Impacts as a Result of Caregiving

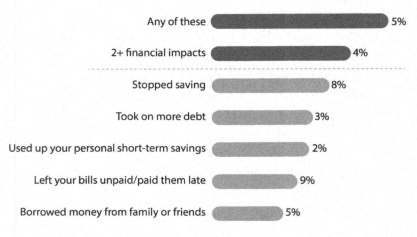

Any of these	5%
2+ financial impacts	4%
Stopped saving	8%
Took on more debt	3%
Used up your personal short-term savings	2%
Left your bills unpaid/paid them late	9%
Borrowed money from family or friends	5%

https://www.aarp.org/content/dam/aarp/ppi/2020/05/full-report-caregiving-in-the-united-states.doi.10.26419-2Fppi.00103.001.pdf
Figure 69 accessed 12/5/2020

"I know Nicole shared it with her brother, Erik. According to the Fidelity Retiree Health Care Cost Estimate, an average retired couple age sixty-five in 2020 may need approximately $295,000 saved after taxes to cover health-care expenses in retirement.[14] For affluent investors, that number can rise to $320,000 or more depending on state taxes.[15] The article warns that many people assume Medicare will cover all health-care costs in retirement, but apparently it doesn't. The article says that about 15 percent of the average retiree's annual expenses will be used for health care-related expenses. It's a pretty eye-opening article, Jodi."[16]

Impacts of Medical Expenses on Retirement

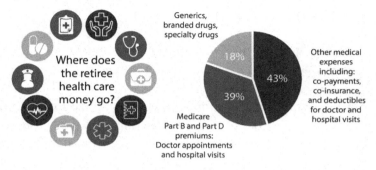

Where does the retiree health care money go?

Generics, branded drugs, specialty drugs — 18%

Other medical expenses including: co-payments, co-insurance, and deductibles for doctor and hospital visits — 43%

Medicare Part B and Part D premiums: Doctor appointments and hospital visits — 39%

How to plan for rising health care costs Estimated cost for health care post-age 65? Try $295,000 per couple in assets needed today. Fidelity Viewpoints 08/03/2020 https://www.fidelity.com/viewpoints/personal-finance/plan-for-rising-health-care-costs accessed 10/10/2020

"I had no idea." Jodi leans in with a concerned look on her face. "That's a big chunk of money."

"Exactly." Jackson nods. "Can you imagine if our own health deteriorates or if we simply have the good fortune, like your parents, to live long enough to experience the effects of aging and then cause this same concern for our children?"

"Yeah," Jodi agrees, "everyone hopes to live a long and healthy life, but it looks like it's going to take some additional planning to stretch our nest egg."

"Honey, Erik and I have been discussing his ability to save for retirement. Since his wife isn't working right now so she can take care of their young kids, it might be tough for a while." Jackson placed another article on the table in front of Jodi. "He shared this with me, knowing you didn't take that promotion because you want more time to help your parents. The article says family caregivers who disrupt their careers or leave the labor force entirely to meet caregiving demands can face substantial

*economic risk and both short- and long-term financial
difficulties."* [17]

*Jackson and Jodi sit quietly at the table consumed by
their thoughts and dreading what lies ahead.*

So many of us, in one way or another, are like the Jones family.
They don't know how to frame the conversation, they don't know the
next steps, and they certainly don't have a plan to deal with what's
coming. Luckily, after listening to her husband and hearing how
concerned her children are, Jodi acknowledges that it is time for the
family to navigate a workable plan.

*Jodi decides that she will visit her parents for an initial
conversation and then schedule a Zoom call with everyone to discuss the next steps. After visiting her parents,
Jodi tells her husband, Jackson, that she understands the
need to include the entire family in the conversation, but
she is concerned about upsetting her parents, particularly
her father, who is still pretending that nothing is wrong.
Jackson comforts his wife and waits until she is ready to
continue the conversation.*

*"OK, Jackson. You and the kids are right." Her expres-
sion shows exhaustion and resignation. "I'll arrange a
Zoom call, but we need to include my father since there
is no point in making decisions or proposing ideas unless
he agrees. Does this sound like a reasonable start?"*

*Jackson holds his wife, who beings to softly cry. "Don't
worry, honey. I know this is difficult, but I think it is
for the best."*

"I know you're right, Jackson. I'm just tired."

The reality is that family conversations about the implications of long-term care planning are taxing and difficult. But the stakes are very high.

Poor family planning creates emergencies. Jodi has been aware of her mother's growing unsteadiness. As we will see, her hesitancy to face the issue lands her parents in the emergency room. What will be the outcome? Will Jodi be one of the 30 percent of caregivers who end up providing care for less than a year,[18] or will it take her away from other family members and events for multiple years? Without family involvement, will they know if Grandma or Grandpa are victims of lottery scams or online fraud?[19] Will they be among the 95 percent of people who say they are willing or want to talk about their end-of-life wishes[20] but don't have a way to do so?

Takeaway:

A lack of planning can have serious consequences for caregivers, impacting their health, happiness, finances, and relationships. A lack of planning often creates two difficult conversations, one with an aging adult and a second with a caregiver in denial.

CHAPTER 7

Setting Up Communication Channels

Good communication is the key to success in any undertaking but especially when dealing across generations. In personally caring for or arranging care for friends or family members, individuals need to be understood, keeping in mind that life experiences differ greatly from one generation to another. Extended or long-term care options that work for one generation may be uncomfortable or unaffordable for another. The Jones family is typical of veiled generational challenges.

The Jones family spans three adult generations, which leaves plenty of room for misunderstanding, misinterpretation, and a lack of actionable knowledge.

Jackson arranges a Zoom call with Erik and Nicole. He invites Jodi's parents to join a bit later than Erik and Nicole so he can bring them up to speed. Greetings indicate that everyone is happy to connect. Despite not wanting to dampen the mood, Jackson moves on to the topic at hand. He tells his children that he shared the information they provided and that Jodi is now on board, acknowledging her parents' growing need for help.

"Mom visited with Grandma and Grandpa. It's true that Grandma Carolyn has slowly become less steady on her feet. Of course, we've all now noticed it. Your mom has been dealing with it for some time. Your grandparents will join us in a few minutes, and we want to be careful to respect that they may not immediately warm to the idea of us arranging a plan for their future care. Let's all remember that God gave us one mouth but two ears for a reason!"

Just then, Jodi interrupts. "Oh, Grandpa is in the waiting room. I'll admit him."

Warm greetings are shared and James announces that Grandma will not be joining. Already very concerned about Grandma, everyone carefully maintains their warm expressions.

Jodi breaks the silence. "Dad, you and I discussed that Grandma is not as steady on her feet as she once was. I did some research and, frankly, I'm alarmed to learn that statistically, when an elderly person falls, their hospital stays are almost two times longer than those of elderly patients who are admitted for any other reason. The risk of falling increases with age and is greater for women than men. Annually, falls are reported by one-third of all people over the age of sixty-five. Two-thirds of those who fall will do so again within six months. Sadly, falls are the leading cause of death from injury among people age sixty-five and older with more than half of all fatal falls involving people age seventy-five or over.[21] Our natural instinct is to avoid the topic of aging, but that simply is not smart."

James, looking concerned, takes a moment to internalize the information, "I had no idea. For Grandma, the most profound effect of falling would be the loss of her ability to function independently." Chuckling, he adds, "or her version of independently."

Wanting to appear supportive of Grandpa's attempt at humor, the family members nod or smile, but it is easy to read their faces, which clearly indicate that they fear that their grandma is at risk of adding to those scary statistics.

Jodi decides that this is her opportunity to be more open with her dad. "And as long as we are discussing this together, let me share that Jackson and I are equally concerned about the effects that Grandma's unsteadiness could have on you, both emotionally and physically, Dad."

Jodi's son, Erik, seizes the opportunity to add, "OK, while we are adding concerns about the effects on Grandpa, we should also discuss the effects it is having on you, Mom."

"Oh, right," Jodi acknowledges with a twinge of discomfort. "I saw the research you and Nicole did on your own concerning the effects of caregiving on the caregiver." Worried that this acknowledgment will upset her father, she hurriedly adds, "However, let's all agree that we need to focus on your grandparents first. We do not

want to wait until Grandma's unsteadiness turns into an emergency."

"Especially with all of us still working." As an after-thought Erik asks, "Who would take care of her?"

"I want to take care of her," James firmly announces, revealing his affection for his wife and his intention to stay in control. Jodi may be the family matriarch, but James certainly sees himself as fiercely independent and as head of his household.

Realizing that her father did not understand Erik's remark as it was intended, Jodi tries to clear up the misunderstanding.

"Dad, can you agree, as remote a chance as it is, that it is possible that you might not be able to take care of Mom as you would wish?" Clearly, her father is struggling with the idea of losing control over where this planning meeting is heading. Hoping to reestablish a caring and open atmosphere, Jodi adds, "That is why we're all on this call, to try to work together to prepare for the unexpected."

Tensions are starting to surface, so the Jones family will have to find a way to move forward and foster a level of cooperation, keeping individual emotions and reactions under control. Planning for care is a multilayered process.

Grandpa James is aware of the toll that helping him and Grandma Carolyn has taken on his daughter. He knows she has taken time off from work and had to pass up a promotion. He has seen what a roller coaster of emotions it has been for both his daughter and his son-in-law.

He also suspects that Jodi has started to put funds aside in case she needs to pay for services or provide other financial assistance. He read an article about the effect it would have on his daughter's retirement if she continues to help them. It saddens him, but until now, he really didn't know what to do about it. Hard as it will be, he agrees to participate in the process since Jodi said it is a just-in-case scenario.

Grandpa James closes the call with a smile, saying, "OK, let's do it." He sees the relief spread over the faces of the others. He experiences a flood of mixed emotions, but he is determined to be supportive—provided he approves of this plan!

There are no hard-and-fast rules for extended or long-term care planning. We know that Grandpa is not necessarily on the same page as the rest of the family. We will see how the Jones family uses my three simple steps to work toward a solution. The steps are a natural progression, similar to what we see during a home renovation. The home represents a family's history and emotional ties for multiple generations. During the renovation's design phase, family values, dreams, and wishes come to light. As things progress, decisions are made based on what is possible since not every wish and want can become a reality. Similarly, the reality of planning for a family's eventual need for limited, extended, or long-term care initially involves the gathering of factual information.

Next, construction begins and inevitably challenges arise. Challenges are overcome by having the right person in the right role. The team works to create the best possible solution. Compromises must be made based on feasible options, priorities, and practicalities, so the team must work together. In the end, the family, advisors, designers, and workers are pretty happy with the results. In each case, the overall process is the same, but the outcomes vary by family needs and resources. In a nutshell, they used a process. The Jones family, like most, need a similar process that leads to accomplishing their goal. And like the home renovation team, both planners and recipients will have to gather information, assign roles, examine options, and accept modifications and changes along the way.

The Jones family will work their way through the three simple steps to create the following:

- A Care Guide
- A Care Squad
- A Care Planning Team

The result will be a practical, funded, personalized plan. These three simple steps allow each person to contribute and participate. No single person will carry the burden of caring for a loved one while juggling their own needs, careers, and home lives. Importantly, Grandpa James will feel that he has a say in finding an option that will work for him and his wife, Carolyn.

Takeaway:

Veiled generational challenges are imbedded in multifaceted, multigenerational planning. The three simple steps provide an *inclusive* rather than *exclusive* approach, with the goal of creating a functioning, effective planning unit.

CHAPTER 8

Step One: Preparing for Immediate or Extended Care Needs

The Care Guide is a collection of important information about an individual, couple, or family. It is filled with relevant, accurate, and up-to-date information for families to offer health-care professionals in case of an emergency. It might contain birthdates, heights, weights, allergies, health conditions, medications (with dosages), primary language, emergency contacts, doctors' and specialists' contact information, and more. If a crisis occurs, no one has to scramble to find information because it's in the Care Guide. This collection of information is a great planning tool. When planning, the more you know about the person you're helping, the better. Even if that person is you!

Creating a Care Guide is a window into the past and a view of the present. The process of gathering documents to create a Care Guide helps you understand what kind of protection is in place and what type of planning they have or have not done. Creating a Care Guide can prompt important conversations and start the extended or long-term care planning ball rolling. It leads to insights that help the family get organized and anticipate future needs.

Here's a list of some basic elements for a Care Guide:

- Basic Questionnaire: The questionnaire should cover health history, family health history (including prior hospital stays), medications (both prescribed and over-the-counter), allergies, primary language, travel exposures, implanted devices, hearing, vision, dental needs, chronic conditions, and any other topics that may impact various medical treatments.
- Professional Contacts Questionnaire: Include the contact information for any doctors, specialists, CPAs, attorneys, advisors, etc.
- Personal Contacts Questionnaire: Include emergency contact information for family, friends, neighbors, and so on.
- Financial Worksheet: Provide information about any investments, insurance, savings, and debts.
- Wishes of Care Recipient Questionnaire
- Legal Questionnaire: Provide information about wills, directives, contracts, beneficiary documents, trusts, etc.
- Medicare, Medicaid, Veterans Questionnaire
- Contract with Caregiver/Facility or Agency Document
- Pre-Retirement and/or Retirement Budget Worksheet
- Final Arrangements Questionnaire
- Choosing a Health-Care Surrogate

Each person in the Jones family has seen or heard something about Grandpa James and Grandma Carolyn's medical or financial information. But does anyone know where various documents are kept? Is the information scattered around their house? Is it in a vault at their bank that only they can access? Are there important documents that have been lost or were never executed? Are they kept on a computer with an undisclosed password? In order to be ready for an emergency and long-term care planning, the Jones family needs to centralize important information and fill in the blanks.

The family begins creating a Care Guide for Grandma and Grandpa Jones so they don't have to guess about finances, health, or treatment history. They are released from carrying the burden of self-doubt about whether they will make the right decisions. The information gathered for the Care Guide is key to creating an appropriate, emotional, physical, and financially affordable family plan for any emergency or extended care need that arises.

On the family's next Zoom gathering, Jodi is pleased that everyone is participating in the conversation. The initial awkwardness seems to be fading and conversations are becoming more productive. Small steps and shared responsibilities are beginning. Jodi regrets that she didn't know about the three simple steps sooner. Her dad seems OK with everything so far.

Jackson, actively supportive, offers an agenda to start the call. "We need to gather and organize information and see which, if any, important documents are missing. While we are helping Grandma and Grandpa get organized, let me also say that this is something we should all prepare for each member of our families. None of us is getting any younger. Aging and accidents happen! It's important to be prepared."

Jodi shoots Jackson a look signaling him to stay focused on Grandma and Grandpa.

"But today our focus is Grandpa James and Grandma Carolyn," Jackson continues. *"First, we need to decide who will handle all their documentation."*

"I will," Nicole volunteers. *"I'll create a spreadsheet with different categories like health history, medications, insurance, and so forth. I'll make sure to add the contact information for their doctors, accountants, and lawyers."*

"Nicole, you are so sweet," Grandpa James says adoringly, *"but I know you are very busy at work."*

"Don't worry, Grandpa, you and Grandma are my favorite project." Nicole blows her grandfather a kiss through her iPad.

"Thank you, Nicole, but we don't want to be a burden. Why don't I just write everything out that you need to know."

"But, Grandpa," Nicole interjects, *"we really need to have everything in one place. We're not trying to be nosy. We're trying to keep you safe."*

"I understand, sweetheart, and I don't want to seem defensive, but there is just certain information that Grandma and I feel is for our eyes only. You know, we've been doing OK handling this all ourselves for a very long time."

"Yes, you have, and I respect that, Grandpa." Nicole leans in. *"But now we have to plan for the future. It's important and it's why we're having this conversation— because we love you. What if you fall and injure yourself*

and Grandma doesn't know how to handle it or doesn't have the information she needs for the hospital? We don't want you or her to become a statistic. We want to help. What if we do this together, Grandpa—the two of us?"

Grandpa James smiles and nods. "I like the compromise." He thinks, but doesn't say out loud, "And you won't need to go through our personal belongings to find what you need."

Thinking back to the statistics his mother shared about falls, Nicole's brother, Erik, weighs in. "Let's start by organizing the information we need to handle any immediate needs that might arise."

The Jones family has navigated the first steps in creating a Care Guide for Grandpa James and Grandma Carolyn. The family explained why they think a Care Guide is important and addressed Grandpa's concerns about privacy and control. They can now begin gathering information and organizing the necessary documents.

The next step is to create a Care Squad to help manage the response in a family emergency. Step Two comes with its own challenges and opportunities. Step One—the Care Guide—is about coming together, organizing, and opening lines of communication. Step Two—the Care Squad—is about creating an action plan and assigning people to each role in that plan. Currently, all roles fall on Jodi's shoulders. She is a pretty typical caregiver, and more and more of us are finding ourselves in that role.

Takeaway:

Getting organized is not everyone's strong suit. The Care Guide provides the framework to organize information and documentation. It benefits both the caregiver's and the care recipient's safety and well-being.

CHAPTER 9

Step Two:
Creating a Care Squad
That Really Cares

According to a November 2019 AARP Public Policy Institute (PPI) report, in 2017 about 41 million unpaid family caregivers provided an estimated 34 billion hours of care—worth $470 billion—to their parents, spouses, partners, and friends. The report explores the growing scope and complexity of caregiving today, which includes an aging population, more family caregivers in the paid workforce, and an increasing amount of medical and nursing tasks that caregivers now provide at home. Family caregivers often experience positive effects and feelings of satisfaction and meaning. But the bigger story is that they typically feel highly strained and overwhelmed.[22]

As a nation, we need to stop pushing this issue to the back burner. In about fifteen years, Americans will have more older relatives or close friends to potentially care for than children. The US Census Bureau projects that, by the year 2035, adults age sixty-five or older will outnumber children under the age of eighteen for the first time in US history.[23]

The 2020 National Alliance for Caregiving report reveals an increase in the number of family caregivers in the United States of 9.5 million from 2015 to 2020. Family caregivers now encompass more than one in five Americans. Alarmingly, the study also reveals that family caregivers have worse health compared to five years ago.[24]

Caught in the sandwich generation, Jodi is typical of most caregivers. She started out offering occasional help to her parents. Gradually, almost unconsciously, her obligations as a caretaker grew as her parents aged. As is often the case, caregivers themselves often slowly become at risk.

Spouses and partners often act as caregivers. Grandpa James seems pretty fit. While filling in the various forms for the Care Guide, the family was reminded that James has a pacemaker, takes medication, and has a family history of heart failure. Despite Jodi's best efforts to limit her father's caregiving role, James, by default, has fast become Carolyn's primary caregiver. James is the *on-site caregiver* and Jodi is the *on-call caregiver*.

Here are some statistics from a recent survey by Cambia Health Solutions:

- 36 percent of caregivers are 18 to 34 years old.
- 62 percent are married or living with their partner.
- Caregivers are almost evenly split between women (53 percent) and men (47 percent).
- 54 percent of caregivers are employed full-time or part-time.
- 58 percent have a child in the household.
- 24 percent of caregivers provide care for both a child (under the age of 18) and an adult (over the age of 18).
- 64 percent of caregivers use at least one digital tool to help manage their caregiving responsibilities.[25]

In the Jones family, between Grandpa James and his caregiver daughter, Jodi, they fall into several of the categories. As is the case in many families, Jodi knows that her husband Jackson's parents may soon need some assistance too. Alarmingly, some of the caregiver statistics include children who are around the same age as Erik and Nicole. If Jodi gets worn out by her caregiving role and needs help, then Erik and/or Nicole will become caught in the sandwich generation and will also add to these statistics. This generational family needs a plan to handle all this!

Creating a Care Squad is a simple but effective step for organizing limited resources. One recommendation for assigning responsibilities is to start with tasks that fit easily into the Care Squad member's current lifestyle. If you live far away but can do finances, that's perfect. If you are available to drive to doctor appointments, volunteer for that. If you can deal with technology as an aid to aging in place, do that. If you live close by, be the one to grab the Care Guide. Find things that work easiest or best with current availability and then move on to things that might be more of an infringement on an individual's schedule.

Additionally, in an emergency, assigned roles help to minimize chaos and hysteria. Finally, knowing they are part of the family Care Squad, family members feel less helpless or excluded.

Let's see how the Jones are doing with moving to Step Two.

"I want to thank all of you for pitching in and getting Step One done!" The family seems pleased with themselves and the relief on Jodi's face is truly a pleasure to see. "Now, let's get started with Step Two. In an emergency or when long-term care is needed, we have all seen responses that are frantic, emotional, unorganized, or disjointed."

"You should hear some of the horror stories my friends share with Grandma and me," Grandpa James says.

Thrown off balance by the looming reality of her father's remark, Jodi regains her composure. "In order to avoid those kinds of reactions in stressful situations, which can only lead to family anxiety and upset, or guilt for not being available and confusion about who should be responsible for what, we will create a Care Squad. This step is not complicated, but it is very effective. One recommendation I have for assigning responsibilities is to start with basic tasks that fit easily into our current lifestyles and then add as needed.

Here is a simple diagram that we can fill in based on everyone's availability and comfort level."

Working together and taking into account each generation's current responsibilities, they create an organized response in case of emergency.

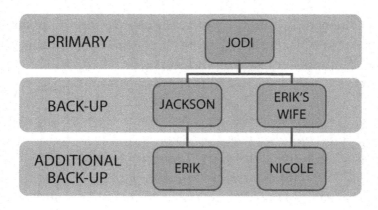

The Jones Family has made good progress. Before they can move on to Step Three, there's an emergency. We get to see Steps One and Two in action.

"Jodi and Jackson take Jodi's parents over to visit with Erik, his wife, and their young children. Happy to have all four generations together, the family sets up chairs outside in the yard. The ground outside is not as level as inside, so Grandma Carolyn's and Grandpa James's chairs are placed on the driveway. Grandma Carolyn, a bit unsteady on her feet, tries to get up and starts to fall. James is sitting next to her and tries to break her fall. They both tumble onto the hard surface of the driveway.

Grandma Carolyn is in a good deal of pain, and Grandpa James seems to have broken his wrist. Both are very pale, and Jodi looks very shaken up. Erik calls for an ambulance. Jackson and Jodi will go with her parents to the hospital. Erik will need to calm the children down. And since both Jodi and Jackson are heading to the hospital, according to the Care Squad chart, Nicole is the backup. She will head to Grandpa James and Grandma Carolyn's house. She knows where the Care Guide is kept and will grab it. She will then head directly to the hospital with the needed information about their insurance, prescriptions, dosages, allergies, previous episodes, health directives, etc.

Grandpa James and Grandma Carolyn, in pain and pretty unhappy, will not have to be further upset by trying to remember essential details and documented information. Three generations pull together and avoid the additional anxiety that comes with facing sudden and unexpected care events.

Once they are back home, Jodi turns to her husband. Expecting a flood of tears, Jackson is surprised to see Jodi composed.

Jodi said, "Well, that went better than I would have ever expected! Everyone seemed to spring into action instead of overdoing it! With Nicole getting and delivering the Care Guide, calling her brother to keep him informed, then bringing us coffee, I was able to concentrate on supporting Mom and Dad. The emergency room took the documents, which helped speed us through the check-in process. Remember last time when we waited and waited while searching for current documents and information. I saw my dad's face when the attending complimented us for being prepared. He assured my parents that with their Care Guide in hand, he could confidently move forward with his assessment and suggested treatment. Although they were in pain, they seemed less scared since the process and care was going along pretty smoothly."

Jackson opened his mouth, shut it, and instead just smiled, nodding his head in agreement. Hating to diminish Jodi's positive assessment, he still felt obligated to add, "Honey, I think we had better move on to Step Three. Your mom is probably not going to recover too quickly. Your dad will have his cast on for a while. They need a long-term care plan."

"Absolutely, Jackson. Too bad we did not get through that last step before this happened."

The Jones family discovered that Step Two was simple but very impactful. The grandparents experienced a more efficient response, which helped them stay calm. The other two generations were able to act quickly without discussing or bickering about who would do what. The emergency room physician was able to address the grandparents' needs without having to deal with hysterical family members.

Younger generations and families that don't have family members nearby may form a Care Squad that is made up of close friends or neighbors who live close by. You may want to share the Care Guide in a sealed envelope or offer a close neighbor or friend instructions on how to find the Care Guide in your home.

Takeaway:

The Care Squad should be practical in assigning roles based on individual schedules and aptitudes in order to use resources efficiently and unburden the on-call, on-site and/or on-a-flight caregivers.

CHAPTER 10

Step Three:
Bringing the Right People to
Your Care Planning Team

The driveway incident was a harsh wake-up call for the Jones family, and many of us can relate. Once the grandparents are released from the hospital, ongoing care will be required. It is a harbinger of future care needs.

Now that the emergency has passed, the members of the Jones family need to get back to their own lives. But now they know they need to prepare for long-term care needs. This is the primary objective of the Care Planning Team (CPT). To accomplish this, it is best to get family or friends to work together toward a solution.

The first issue is, who should be invited to participate in a Care Planning Team? The Jones family includes three adult generations, all of whom are absorbed by their own busy lives. Nicole is very engaged in her career; Erik is the sole support of his family; Jodi is already busy supervising her mother's recovery, settling her father into a new routine, and trying to keep her job (she has given up the idea of a promotion); and Jackson, working full-time, has concerns about his own parents, who are starting to need some guidance and help. In addition, getting Grandpa James to cooperate is still a challenge. Let's see how they handle it.

> *"Well, we dodged that bullet." Jodi says, sitting alone with Jackson. She still isn't fully recovered from the bad fright. Her initial reaction, appreciating the effectiveness of Steps One and Two, has given way to the reality of having her parents return to their home. "Mom is doing OK but has a pretty intense recovery road ahead of her. Dad has a cast that I am sure he will have the kids sign!" She nervously laughs.*
>
> *Jackson replies, "Thank goodness we were able to spring into action. The Care Guide alone solved lots of potential problems." He briefly pauses. "What I liked best about the Care Squad was it minimized having too many helping hands, which let others do what they needed to do." Reaching over, Jackson puts his hand gently on his wife's shoulder. "Honey, I hope you agree that there is no way you can be the only one helping your parents as they heal. We will now certainly have to get them some in-home help."*
>
> *"I know, I know!" Rubbing her temples, Jodi says, "I worry that they will reject the idea as an invasion of their privacy and try to handle things on their own."*
>
> *Seeing his wife so tense and worried, Jackson flatly states, "Well, that is not really a viable option."*

Worried about her parents' reaction to a team approach, Jodi doesn't jump right into Step Three. Jackson eases his wife into the idea that they need to explore viable options as soon as possible.

Rather than have Jodi try to do everything alone, even with some help from her husband, a Care Planning Team would allow the family to work together to investigate, research, and work with agents, advisors, or specialists to secure viable options. In establishing the CPT, be as inclusive as possible. Exclusivity can stir up a family feud.

Let me share a personal story with you. It was a tough lesson. My husband's parents nominated their older son, my husband, as their executor. They didn't include their younger son in the planning process. My husband's father passed away, leaving the two sons to care for their mother. During the time that their mother lived in an assisted living facility (ALF) and later when she was required to move into the nursing home (NH) wing of the facility, the two of them continually argued about who should be in charge of their mother's care, what facility was best, and all sorts of related cost-of-care issues. Emotions run high when dealing with someone else's care: love, guilt, hope, fear, confusion, worry, along with a myriad of other emotions can quite often manifest into a family feud. To this day, the brothers do not speak to each other or their wives and children. It is and remains a divided family. I am sure it isn't what his parents would have wanted, and I am certain that if they had created a CPT they may have argued, but both brothers and their families would have felt heard and would forcibly have worked toward a compromise. Not inviting a family member (or close friend where appropriate) to be part of the CPT is the same as excluding them. Explain the role and time commitment. If they cannot find the time to participate in the CPT, it is wise to let them indicate as much. If during the process they decide to drop out, you still are not the one who excluded them.

In my experience, since not every family member may be as cooperative as one might hope, the CPT must establish some commonsense rules. Each individual and each generation has its own vocabulary and is influenced by its own lifestyle, value system, and maturity level. Once the CPT is created, defining and establishing respect for one another should be the main goal. The CPT may have to establish what is on the table and what is off the table. Being included in the CPT is not a license to be intrusive.

Let's see how the Jones family worked out this challenge.

> *"OK," Jodi concedes. "We will ask the kids, and if they say yes, we can ask them to qualify their yes with how much time they can offer."*

> *Furrowing her brow, Jodi expresses one of her real concerns. "But you know my dad will not want to share too many details about his health, and he absolutely will not want to talk about his personal financial information."*

> *Jackson thinks for a couple of minutes. "Then we include everyone in the research, but when it comes to the final decision, you just talk with your dad and his advisors. As CPT members, we participate in the research and discussions, which means we will be better able to understand why a particular option is eliminated or kept for further consideration. We will see how eligibility requirements and the funding of various options play a role in the planning process. You let the kids know that when it comes to a final decision, an advisor or two will be involved to help your parents determine the most feasible option to create the most workable long-term care plan."*

> *"You're right. You're right!" Jodi is ecstatic with relief at Jackson offering a practical arrangement so they can move forward. "OK, we continue with all three*

*generations participating with a degree of privacy to keep
Dad comfortable."*

"And cooperative," Jackson mutters.

As it turns out, both Nicole and Erik do want to be included. Rather than drive the family members apart, although they may disagree or argue during the process, ultimately, they will at least accept the solution or, better yet, feel a bond by helping to arrange for the safety and care of their grandparents and, by extension, their mother, Jodi.

Takeaway:

Be inclusive but not naive. Establish some rules. In the absence of a natural leader, consider an advisor as a facilitator or mediator so the planning process doesn't stall.

CHAPTER 11

Figuring Out a Budget without Tearing Your Family Apart

Now that the Jones family has established their CPT members, another major element is affordability. To be sustainable, the plan must work with the current budget, but of equal importance, the plan must work with a future budget. Life events, such as unemployment, births, deaths, divorce, retirement, and so on, all need to be considered.

In order to know what is feasible in terms of a general financial commitment, it is helpful, if not necessary, to get a grasp on the present-day costs for various care facilities and in-home services. There are several costs of care studies and tools that major insurers and associations offer.[26] These sites show how the cost of care varies based on the care setting, geographic location, and level of care required, among other things. Although most people recognize that the cost for health care continually increases, it is not unusual to experience sticker shock when you see actual and projected costs for extended or long-term care.

What is especially engaging and enlightening about these geographical cost-of-care studies is that you can enter various cost percentage increases (like 3 percent or 4 percent) to get estimates of future costs five to thirty years into the future. This provides a good barometer of the direction costs may head. Seeing the rate of increasing costs aids in formulating a plan that is not only realistic in the present but sustainable for the long haul.

One insurer included a follow-up study focused on the drivers of the cost of care.[27] This research, done prior to the full impact of the pandemic, certainly agrees with what we witnessed during COVID-19. The following factors continue to contribute to increasing costs:

- Labor shortages
- Personal protective equipment (PPE) costs
- Regulatory changes (including updated CDC guidelines)
- Employee recruitment and retention challenges
- Wage pressures
- Supply and demand

This is instructional but also very sobering information. It has the same effect on the Jones family.

> *They are screen-sharing on their Zoom call and reviewing costs by manipulating the cost-of-care study tool. After a lively discussion about the drivers of the cost of care, the Jones family lapses into a pensive silence.*
>
> *Nicole breaks the silence by sharing a conversation that she had with her cousin. "Our cousin Tyson, who is a first responder, volunteered for extra work shifts during the pandemic. He shared some really heartbreaking stories about the personal effect that the shortage of qualified medical and nonmedical workers had on not just patients but also his buddies and their families. Watching family*

members look frantic and sick people look terrified was awful. Think of how many of them have no plan, no idea of what to do over the long-term for someone they care about who survived the ordeal or simply is no longer comfortable living on their own. You would think more people would now consider doing some extended and long-term care planning."

"You know" Erik says, picking up his sister's thread, "during the pandemic, we were sort of forced to follow a plan. Wearing masks, distancing from others, washing our hands, getting vaccinated, and generally being aware of and following Center of Disease Control (CDC) guidelines became a universal guide/plan. Countries and states that were able to follow the plan were not as hard hit as those that did not. Can you imagine the cost of the care? It makes the rising costs of health care seem more understandable. While others may not see the necessity to plan for long-term or extended health-care costs, we sure do. We need an affordable, practical plan to keep our grandparents safe for the long haul."

Grandpa James, happy to become the center of his grandchildren's affection, laughingly teases, "Let's hope Grandma and I are in it for the long haul."

"You have to be," Erik responds, smiling broadly, "since we are all planning for it. And plans work!"

Dispelling the sadness left by the realities of the pandemic and Grandma's medical scare, and recognizing the importance of planning, the CPT is ready to start learning about some of the basic costs associated with different care options. Turning his attention back to the cost of

*care chart that Jodi still has up on her screen, Erik asks,
"What's the difference between a home care aide and
home health aide?"*

Genworth Cost of Care 2020

Category	2004 Cost	2020 Cost	Total Increase ($)	Average Annual Increase ($)	Total Percent Increase ($)
Private Room Nursing Home	$65,185	$105,850	$40,665	$2,542	62.38%
Assisted Living Facility	$28,800	$51,600	$22,800	$1,425	79.17%
Home Care Home Health Aide	$42,168	$54,912	$12,744	$797	30.22%
Home Care Homemaker	$38,095	$53,763	$15,673	$980	41.14%

Represents average cost through 2008, switched to median in 2009. Genworth Cost of Care Survey 2004-2020, Conducted by CareScout*
** United States Department of Labor, Bureau of Labor Statistics opens in new window, Accessed 11/08/20
https://www.genworth.com/aging-and-you/finances/cost-of-care/cost-of-care-trends-and-insights.html

Erik's question is important. Specialized definitions and terminology should be clarified. In most cases, answers can often be found, as in this case, right on the website.

> *Jodi reads aloud. "A home care aide refers to nonclinical
> help, such as meal prep and companionship, while home
> health aides, or they may be called patient care assistants,
> help with daily activities such as cleaning, bathing, toi-
> leting, dressing, housekeeping, scheduling, transferring,
> shopping for groceries, and serving meals. If qualified,
> some home health aides can check vital signs such as
> pulse, temperature, and respiration rate."*

At this stage, they may need to get advice from a professional. For example, aside from the basic information, when it comes to in-home care, there is a minimum number of hours for which you can hire either one. There may be added travel or other costs as well. There is also the issue of deciding if you want to engage an agency, who does background checks, certifications or insurance, and so forth.

Grandma won't be in the hospital for long. The family needs to quickly figure out which options work for long-term care needs. They get organized by first creating a simple summary of facts.

Takeaway:

Accessing websites and utilizing tools to better understand current and future costs for various levels and settings of care, as well as knowing how to evaluate in-home or facility care options, is essential for working toward a sustainable financial plan.

CHAPTER 12

A Simple Summary Highlights Immediate Actions

F or the sake of privacy and efficiency, it is important that only necessary information, relevant to considering various options, be presented in a summary format to the CPT. The Care Guide is a good resource for creating a quick summary from which the CPT can work.

How does the list look for Grandma and Grandpa Jones family? Behind the scenes, Jodi worked with her father, James, to put a basic summary together.

"Hi everyone, thanks for joining. In order to move forward, let me share a summary that Grandpa and I put together using family history and information from several of the Care Guide questionnaires and worksheets. Thanks to Nicole for the work she did with Grandpa. This summary will help us as we consider and eliminate

various limited, extended, or long-term care options. At the end of the process, it will help us explain to specialists why certain options appeal to Grandma and Grandpa."

Jodi presents the following summary:

- *Grandpa is a veteran.*
- *Grandpa receives social security benefits.*
- *Grandma also receives spousal social security benefits.*
- *Their income is supplemented by a modest amount from savings and investments.*
- *They are very proud to say that they have no mortgage on their home, which has increased in value over the thirty years they have lived in it.*
- *They both have Medicare and Medicare Advantage policies.*
- *Grandpa has a Whole Life insurance policy, but as you all know, he has stated unequivocally that beneficiary proceeds are to be equally divided between his grandchildren, Erik and Nicole.*
- *They drew up a will, but it has not been updated for many years.*
- *Neither of them has an advance medical directive, a durable power of attorney for health care or property, or a do-not-resuscitate order.*

A quick review of the summary indicates that the grandparents should immediately take care of important legal documents. They would be well advised to update their will and create legal medical directives. Family and/or close friends prefer to know someone's wishes in case of illness, mental incapacity, or a prolonged inability to properly make health-care decisions. Each state has specific regulations and forms available for use. If done correctly, these directives and documents save the family, friends, and professionals a great deal of difficulty and angst by providing guidance. If someone changes their state of residency, it is important to see if new documents are needed. There is a helpful site [28] to identify and locate elder and special needs law attorneys. The site is searchable by attorney name, practice area, language, or zip code.

If you don't know the zip codes for nearby towns where your parents or friends live (or maintain a legal residence) or the area to which they plan to retire, the site offers a link to look up a location's zip code. Once the documents and directives are in good order, duplicates should be added to the Care Guide.

Once the summary is complete and immediate documentation needs are identified, the CPT can move on to long-term care needs. It makes for a more interesting exercise when each member's assignment relates to their own potential planning needs. However, the Jones family must make the grandparents their first priority since time is not on their side.

Takeaway:

No one wants to make life and care decisions for others without some guidance. Step Three opens conversations that help determine whether up-to-date documentation (or at the very least any notes) concerning wishes and preferences is available.

CHAPTER 13

Build a Knowledge Base about Long-Term Care Options

Although they feel some pressure to hurry and find a long-term solution for the grandparents, the CPT still needs to consider options that will last as long as the need. The discovery of nonexistent and outdated important documents during Step One has already been very beneficial to the CPT.

Let's see how more than one generation benefits as they review the grandparents' summary.

> *Caregiver Jodi's tone has gone from overwrought to encouraged to cautiously upbeat. "Hello everyone. I am happy to report that we got the necessary documentation done and found a local estate planner to update the wills." Looking pleased, she pauses and then proudly announces, "Dad and I realized that we also were missing some important documents. We worked with the same*

firm and created missing documents for ourselves as well! None of you will be asked to make decisions for us without knowing our preferences."

Erik says, "My wife and I updated our wills after the birth of our daughter. We are not planning any additions to the family, so we hope this will serves us well for a long, long time."

Erik's remark brings on some family teasing about having another child. Grandpa starts to relax as he sees the process is not focused only on him and his wife, Carolyn.

Erik, laughing along with the CPT, tries to redirect the group. "Mom assigned us different options to look into. Who has long-term care insurance?"

As the CPT investigates different options for the grandparents, they will discover that many long-term care options do not involve insurance. However, traditional long-term care (TLTC) insurance is often the popular suggestion. If the option seems to fit, they will engage an agent or advisor for a more in-depth review.

Traditional Long-Term Care (TLTC) Insurance

Jodi starts with an overview of TLTC. "I looked at traditional long-term care insurance. I discovered that there are at least three basic issues to consider for Grandpa James and Grandma Carolyn. Let me share my screen so you can see my summary.

"The first issue is suitability. Is the insurance product appropriate for them, based on their goals and financial situation? The second issue is underwriting. Will they

qualify based on their past and current health status? The third issue is affordability and sustainability. Can they pay current and future premiums?

Like life insurance, the initial price of a long-term care insurance policy is age sensitive. At their ages, and given their past and current health conditions, if my parents were offered a policy, it is not likely to be affordable."

Nicole candidly asks, "So where do we go from here?"

That's a great question, and it's a pretty common one. Sadly, many people are quick to dismiss finding a solution if the first option doesn't fit. In Step Three, you examine multiple options.

Is self-funding a smart option for Grandma Carolyn and Grandpa James given their growing care needs and advancing age? From information gathered for their Care Guide, we know that at least statistically, there is a likelihood that at least one of the grandparents will live into their eighties or beyond. We also know that they have made it very clear that they paid off their mortgage so they could age at home. They have no interest in moving, no matter how lovely the facility may be!

Self-Funding Extended or Long-Term Care Expenses

Currently, medical costs are estimated to consume about 15 percent of an average retiree's annual expenses.[29] If we add a future estimate for long-term care costs, the complications of market timing, liquidity, and the potential for exhausting spousal lifestyle or care funds, self-funding can be a risky proposition.

From the summary, we know that Grandma Carolyn and Grandpa James have been good savers. They also need additional care to begin right away. So, in their case, self-funding does not appear to be a bad option. But a closer look at their financial questionnaire (completed during Step One) reveals a red flag. Like so many of their generation, the grandparents rely heavily on social security benefits to supplement their investment and savings income.

Social Security

When Social Security was launched in 1935, to qualify for full retirement benefits, you had to be sixty-five years old. Back then, you could say that the actuaries got it right since the average life expectancy was sixty-two years. However, expectancies have steadily increased, resulting in a financially stressed system. Additional changes to the Social Security program are likely.

Currently, full retirement age (FRA) is increasing incrementally from sixty-six years to sixty-seven years.[30] The FRA is likely to be pushed further out. However, currently a worker may begin receiving social security retirement benefits as early as age sixty-two. By claiming before full retirement age, monthly benefits will be permanently reduced by as much as 30 percent.

There are many aspects of the Social Security program that we could cover, but that is beyond the scope of this overview. There are numerous websites, articles, and specialists available for personalized advice.

Does relying on social security income impact the grandparents' self-funding option?

> *Grandpa James is sharing some information, sending a signal of cooperation to the CPT. "Your Mom and I spoke with a Social Security specialist. Since Social Security benefits make up a good portion of our income, there is reason to be concerned that we could outlive our current income if it is depleted too quickly by paying for extended home care."*

Grandpa James wants to be clear that it isn't about a lack of good budgeting. In his mind, as part of the silent generation, it's just the way the system works. Not wanting to share details of his own income, he offers a general example.

"Let me share the simple example your mom and I saw. Let's say my current social security monthly income is $3,000 and as my spouse, Grandma receives $1,500. In this example, Grandma receives a spousal benefit based on my work record. She claims at her full retirement age, so her benefit is half of my full retirement age benefit of $3,000. But when one spouse passes away, the other one is left with a diminished social security income to cover living expenses plus extended or long-term care expenses."

Quickly shifting the conversation at the mention of her parents passing away, Jodi encourages the CPT to learn more on their own. "You each should access the Social Security website to create an account. Make sure your personal information and work history is accurately recorded. The site also offers a calculator that lets you enter in various amounts, dates, and so on, to estimate what you may expect to receive when you qualify for social security benefits."[31]

Together, the CPT concludes that given the prospect of their potential longevity, limited savings, and dependency on dual social security income available to cover escalating care costs, self-funding their extended or long-term care is not a viable option for Grandpa James and Grandma Carolyn.

Grandpa James suddenly interjects, reminding everyone that he is very much engaged in this planning exercise and has his priorities. "Before we move on, I promised your grandma that I would remind everyone that Grandma and I want a plan that doesn't burden Jodi or Jackson—or any of you for that matter—with bills for our care. Jodi and Jackson love spoiling their grandchildren, our great-grandchildren. We are so pleased that they started a savings fund for them. Funding our care would interrupt, if not end, that heartfelt gesture."

"What kind of a savings plan?" Nicole asks, glancing around at the others. "Can I contribute too?"

Resource Allocation Challenges

"We opened a 529 plan for them," Jackson explains, "529 plans, legally known as qualified tuition plans, are sponsored by states, state agencies, or educational institutions. The name comes from Section 529 of the Internal Revenue Code. If you start early, as we did, it is an excellent vehicle to fund education costs. We investigated other vehicles, such as money saved in a Roth IRA, a custodial UGMA, or an UTMA account, which can be used for purposes other than education. We did a comparison[32] and decided on a 529 plan. We liked that a 529 plan can be used for graduate school, not just undergraduate school, and depending on state law, may be passed on to the next generation. There is also no age limit on contributions to a 529 plan."

"So you can see, Nicole," Grandpa says, nodding a thanks to Jackson, "my concern here is that if your parents need *to contribute to our care, it could very well interfere not only with funding the 529 plan but also with their other plans as well, such as their retirement plans."*

As a result of using the three simple steps, the Jones family is establishing good avenues of communication. For Grandpa James, as proud as he is of being independent, he realizes that self-funding and traditional insurance options will not work for him and Grandma Carolyn. As a result of working with the CPT to create the Care Guide and establish his Care Squad, without resentment or anger, he reaches that conclusion in sync with his family.

Additionally, the discussion about the 529 plan is a perfect example of how open dialogue leads to more family cohesiveness. While not directly connected to the need for an extended care solution, now everyone understands how the lack of a financially sound care plan could negatively influence the success of the 529 plan or his daughter's retirement plan.

Time to move on to another option that may work for the grandparents. Hopefully, there will be no more red flags!

Takeaway:

Using books and tools to build a knowledge base can translate into choices while avoiding misinformation and miscalculations in funding retirement and extended care planning.

CHAPTER 14

Government Programs: What's the Deal with Medicaid and Medicare?

Viewed through the generational lens of various CPT members, some options seem like a good fit. The prospective care recipient may view things differently. The COVID-19 pandemic demonstrated that aging in a care facility is definitely not on everyone's bucket list. With telehealth and wearable health tracking devices becoming more mainstream, some health-care companies are considering the inclusion or expansion of various home health-care benefits in Medicare Advantage programs. States are also reviewing the home health-care benefits available to Medicaid beneficiaries.

> *Erik, unfamiliar with the ins and outs of government programs, brings up Medicare and Medicaid as possible options. "According to the summary, Grandma and Grandpa both have Medicare and Medicare Advantage plans. Or maybe they qualify for Medicaid?"*

The Medicare and Medicare Basics[33]

Medicare covers medically necessary acute care, such as doctor visits, prescription drugs, and hospital stays. Except for specific circumstances, Medicare does not pay for most long-term care services or personal care, such as help with bathing or for supervision, which is considered custodial care.[34] Medicare does not provide long-term care coverage or custodial care unless medical care is needed.

Medigap plans are intended to fill the "gaps" in Medicare insurance. However, even the most comprehensive Medigap plans do not cover long-term care needs. These policies currently do not pay for assisted living, Alzheimer's disease, custodial care, personal care, or adult day care.[35]

Medicare Advantage plans generally cover specialized care, such as stays in a skilled nursing facility, hospice, respite care, and eligible home health services. Some Medicare Advantage plans now cover certain long-term care and at-home care services.[36]

Recent Changes

Medicare provides benefit payments for three broad categories of treatment: hospital (emergencies and surgeries), medical (doctors and treatments), and pharmaceutical (medicines). Unlike Medicaid, Medicare is an entitlement program, meaning that everyone who reaches age sixty-five and is entitled to receive social security benefits also receives Medicare. Medicare also covers people of any age who are permanently disabled or who have end-stage renal disease. Medicare is financed by multiple tax-funded trust funds, trust fund interest, beneficiary premiums, and additional money approved by Congress.[37]

Medicaid, on the other hand, is a public assistance program that helps pay medical costs for individuals with limited income and assets. To be eligible for Medicaid coverage, you must meet the program's strict income and asset guidelines. The Medicaid program is jointly funded by the federal government and states. The federal government pays states for a specified percentage of program expenditures, called the Federal Medical Assistance Percentage (FMAP).[38] The most significant difference between Medicare and Medicaid in the realm of long-term care planning, however, is that Medicaid covers some of the costs of nursing home care, while Medicare, for the most part, does not."[39] Recent changes in the Centers for Medicare and Medicaid Services rules allow some expansion of long-term services and supports (LTSS) into Medicare Advantage (MA) Plans (also known as Part C Plans) for enrollees. The 2019–2020 expansion of LTSS falls under

Jodi looks a bit sheepish as she responds. "Your grandparents don't like the idea of the government controlling their care options."

"Medicaid is a welfare program," adds Grandpa James. He is not in the least bit sheepish and wants to be sure everyone understands how strongly he feels about this option. "We

Medicare Advantage (Part C) Plans but not under the original Medicare program despite other changes that took effect on January 1, 2020.

Medicare and Medicaid programs are not only complex but also administered by individual states, so it is important to get state-specific answers.

don't qualify, we don't want to qualify, and we don't expect to access a government assistance program. It's for people who haven't been as lucky as us. We worked hard for what we have. We don't want to have to spend or give away what we have in order to qualify for government assistance."

He pauses a moment for emphasis.

"Also, my friends tell me that the process is complicated and the ongoing paperwork will probably have to be handled with the help of a family member. And worst of all, you lose control over your choices."

Not exactly understanding his grandpa's reaction, Erik thinks back to what their mom shared about how his grandparents' generation was impacted by events very different from his own.

Nicole is also a bit surprised by the forcefulness of Grandpa James's response. However, she wants to respect different viewpoints. "Got it, Grandpa," she says.

Seeing everyone nodding their heads, it takes Grandpa James a moment to absorb the support. A smile starts to cross his face as he looks at each one of the people that he loves who accept his opinion, whether they agree or not.

Erik brings up a topic about which he knows his grandpa is proud. "I saw on the summary that Grandpa is a veteran. Dad, you're also a vet. Can Grandpa use VA benefits for long-term care needs?"

"Both Grandpa and I are veterans, but I suspect we qualify for different levels of benefits. I contacted Dan, who specializes in veteran benefits. I consulted him concerning veteran benefits for both Grandpa and myself. Grandpa and I will do a detailed review with him to determine if Grandpa is entitled to any benefits, what is involved in accessing benefits, and if those benefits can change over time. He has the most exhaustive resource list that you can imagine."

Glad to finally hear about an option that may be helpful, the CPT agrees to investigate another option that allows the grandparents to age in their own home. Jodi mentions a friend who has parents in a similar situation and says they were able to secure some funding for long-term care expenses through a reverse mortgage. There is dead silence. The positive vibe disappears. The reactions are anything but positive.

Takeaway:

Each generation filters information based on how and when they acquire it. The CPT overview discovery process helps to avoid assigning solutions that appeal to one generation but not necessarily to another, especially since options change and evolve over time.

CHAPTER 15

The Home as a Funding Solution for Aging in Place

The Jones family's reaction to the mention of a reverse mortgage is by no means unusual. Historically, largely relegated as a product of last resort for the financially infirm, work done by the Academy for Home Equity in Financial Planning at the University of Illinois Urbana-Champaign elevated the status of reverse mortgage lending. Changes made by the Federal Housing Authority (FHA) in 2014 to the Home Equity Conversion Mortgage (HECM) further solidified reverse mortgages as a financial planning tool. The home as an asset for retirement income planning and as a funding solution for aging in place has gained acceptance. This means that home equity, roughly two-thirds of the average American's net worth, is no longer dismissed out of hand in the planning process.

Many individuals fear they risk losing the home if they elect this option. The Jones family is no exception.

Jodi continues their previous discussion. "Hi! Well, we are certainly learning a good deal as Grandma and Grandpa's Care Planning Team!" *However, when Jodi brings up the idea of a reverse mortgage again, Jodi's father immediately becomes alarmed and upset.*

"I am proud to say that Grandma and I do not have a mortgage on our home. We do not want to lose the house to a bank or have you owe a bunch of money to repay any sort of mortgage when we are both gone."

Confused, almost tearing up, and looking around for support from the CPT, Nicole blurts out, "I want to keep my grandparents' house in the family. I have such wonderful memories of holidays and summertime at their house."

Erik adds more generational color to the family's attachment. "Every time I say we are going over to Grandma Carolyn's house, my daughter rubs her belly and says, "Yay! Grandma's house smells good. How many of Grandma's yummy cupcakes can I have?"

Grandpa James, looking very touched, says, "I will mention that to Grandma. She will be very pleased!"

Jodi comments, "I understand everyone's reaction. Actually, I initially had the same reaction. But now there are reverse mortgages that stipulate that no borrower can ever owe more than the value of the house regardless of how long the occupant lives or what housing values do. It's sometimes referred to as a no-negative equity guarantee. It protects the borrower and their estate from being obligated to provide additional resources to cover *the debt. However, we do need to maintain the house and pay the taxes."*

Grandpa James puffs up his chest without realizing the gesture isn't visible from the angle of the Zoom window. He states quite firmly, "We are steadfast in those areas!"

"How do they figure out how much money Grandpa can get?" Nicole asks, reminding everyone that the devil is in the details!

"My understanding," says Jodi, "is that the lender establishes a loan-to-value ratio for the house. Funding is based on the characteristics of the house and the age of the borrower. I invited a specialist to join our call in a couple of minutes. She can offer us advice and answer any questions we may have. Let me admit her."

"Hello everyone, my name is Shelley, and I would like to share some information with you, answer questions, address concerns, and set up a follow-up call. First let me offer you an overview of reverse mortgages and, at the conclusion of our time together, I hope we will be able to use the diagram that I am sharing on my screen to help you decide if this works for your family's needs."

Reverse Mortgage Decision Tree by Shelly Giordano

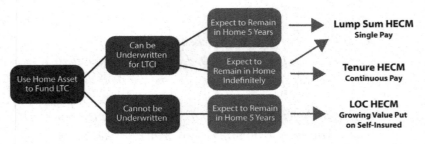

© Shelley Giordano, http://fundinglongevitytaskforce.com What's the deal with…Reverse Mortgages? Second edition, published by People Tested (http://peopletested.com)

Takeaway:

It is in your best interest to truly understand a resource that may have been previously dismissed but now may present a good option.

CHAPTER 16

Putting the Plan in Place: Multiple Options Fit the Bill!

I t was unlikely that the grandparents' income and savings and their burdened caregiver would remain sufficient. After considering multiple options, the CPT soon recognized that government welfare and insurance options were not suitable and/or viable in this case. Instead, the CPT engaged professional guidance to examine and mull over Medicare plan benefits and veteran benefits. In the end, open discussion, research, and respect made it possible to focus on options that worked for the grandparents and to fulfill the grandparents' wish to age in place in the home they love.

Jodi is no longer caught in the shifting of generational responsibilities, where she becomes the parent and her parents become the children. An incredible burden has been lifted. Everyone feels more stable, more hopeful, and more settled with a workable plan in place. The CPT—particularly Grandpa James and Jodi—avoided generational stress, discord, caregiver burnout, and financial hardship by engaging at various levels and at various times in my three simple steps. They created a tailored generational family plan.

The exercise left Jodi wondering if there were additional options available for her, knowing she would one day, hopefully, benefit from a long life and need care.

Takeaway:

Like the Jones family, your family should personalize the three simple steps to start the conversation, understand family dynamics, become educated, and engage with professionals to secure a plan. The three simple steps lead a family to a healthier, more financially secure, and peaceful place.

Veteran Benefits

The organization responsible for veterans' health care:
- VA (1930–1989) Veterans Administration
- VA (1989–present) Department of Veterans Affairs, VA Central Office (VACO)

The Department of Veterans Affairs (VA) delivers a wide array of benefits and services to eligible veterans, dependents, and survivors to help ease the transition from the military to civilian life and to improve quality of life. These programs are overseen by three administrations:

- The Veterans Health Administration (VHA) provides healthcare and pharmacy services.
- The Veterans Benefits Administration (VBA) provides compensation and pension disability benefits, education assistance, life insurance, vocational rehabilitation/employment services, and home loan guaranty assistance.
- The National Cemetery Administration (NCA) provides memorial benefits, including graves, markers, flags, medallions, and burial allowances.

Some veterans have gone years without even realizing their dependents are eligible for benefits.

- Spouses and dependents of a permanently and totally disabled vet can qualify for health insurance through the VA's Civilian Health and Medical Program, or CHAMPVA.

- For veterans who need more help at home, there's a hidden benefit known as the Veteran-Directed Care Program. Veterans participating in this program are able to hire family and friends to provide for their personal care needs, or to provide support to their family caregivers. It authorizes a monthly flexible spending budget.
- For long-term care, the Aid and Attendance benefit is aimed at helping older veterans and their spouses when they can no longer handle daily living tasks, such as dressing and showering, on their own.
- There are also state VA benefits, from exemptions for local property taxes to free fishing and hunting licenses.
- The VA can help with some burial expenses, and it provides a free headstone or marker and burial flag. The VA created a program that allows veterans to apply for burial benefits in advance, so veterans and their families can plan ahead.
- State benefits range from free college and employment resources to free hunting and fishing licenses. Most states also offer tax breaks for their veterans and specialized license plates.

Stats

The largest living cohort of male veterans served during the Vietnam War (August 1964 to April 1975) while the largest living cohort of female veterans served during the post-9/11 period (September 2001 or later). Currently almost all veteran beneficiaries age 65 or older (98 percent) are men.

Data: https://www.va.gov/vetdata/
Data maps: https://www.va.gov/vetdata/Maps.asp
Data FAQ: https://www.va.gov/vetdata/faqs.asp
Statista on veterans: https://www.statista.com/topics/1279/veterans/
Census Bureau on veterans: https://www.census.gov/topics/population/veterans.html
State summaries: https://www.va.gov/vetdata/stateSummaries.asp
National Center for Veterans Analysis and Statistics: https://www.va.gov/vetdata/veteran_population.asp

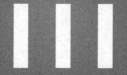

A Growing Marketplace Offers Expanding Options and Planning Tools

CHAPTER 17

The Sandwich Generation Issue Solved—Or Is It?

The Jones family achieved a level of harmony while working together as a team, which initially started as a desire to save Jodi, who is caught in the sandwich generation, from becoming overwhelmed.

Who qualifies as a member of the sandwich generation? According to Pew Research, members of the sandwich generation are mostly middle-aged: 71 percent of members are ages forty to fifty-nine, 19 percent are younger than age forty, and 10 percent are age sixty or older. Men and women are equally likely to be members of the sandwich generation. [41]

Relationships are a key element to an individual's well-being throughout their life span. [42] But whether it is work, education, marriage or the dissolution of a marriage or partnership, military service, or travel, distance exacerbates the challenges of being caught in the sandwich generation. Another popular expression for this upside-down responsibility is *role reversal*. The child must take on the role of the parent. Psychologically, let alone physically or financially, this is not an easy task.

As we saw with the Jones family, becoming caught in the sandwich generation typically starts with just "helping out." A chore here or there. Gradually, caregiver responsibilities increase along with care needs. Since it appears that you are handling things, other family members or friends may not even be aware or want to acknowledge the impact it is having on both you and the care recipient. Sharing Jodi's story as she and her family move through the three simple steps is a way to introduce the topic and suggest a way to formulate a plan.

Let's check back in to see how the Jones family is doing now that Jodi and Jackson, while still part of the sandwich generation, are no longer experiencing the many negative and unwanted challenges brought about by the absence of a plan for the grandparents' well-being.

Jodi is looking and feeling much better now that her parents are secure and have a plan that they are comfortable with and can afford, but most importantly, allows them to age at home. Jackson is happy that his wife is able to enjoy a more normal work/life balance and now has time to do some fun things with him and their grandchildren. Jodi arranges a CPT wrap-up call, minus her dad, to remind everyone that they will periodically review Grandpa James and Grandma Carolyn's plan.

Despite her father's reluctance and sometimes forceful remarks, utilizing the three simple steps pulled this family together instead of apart. But she will not soon forget how unaware she was of the effect her caregiver duties was having on other generations.

Generational Implications Create a Redo

Jodi is motivated to pay it forward. "Hey, honey, take a look at this."

Jackson leans over and looks at Jodi's iPad. "What am I seeing?"

"Look at his chart; it shows that according to estimates from the US Census Bureau, millennials have surpassed baby boomers as the nation's largest living adult generation."

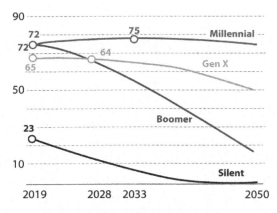

Projected Population by Generation
(In Millions)

Note: Millennials refer to the population ages 23 to 38 as of 2019.
Source: Pew Research Center tabulationsof U. S. Cenus Bureau population estimates released April 202 and population projections released December 2017.

Source: Richard Fry. "Millennials overtake Baby Boomers as America's largest poplulation", Pew Research Center, April 28, 2020.
https://www.pewresearch.org/fact-tank/2020/04/28/millennials-overtake-baby-boomers-as-americas-largest-generation/

"Really? We have been displaced!" Jackson jokes, but he clearly isn't sure where Jodi is going with this conversation.

"Millennials will be between ages twenty-five and forty in 2021, and GenXers will be ages forty-one to fifty-six. In 2019, millennials numbered 72.1 million and GenXers are projected to pass baby boomers in population by 2028."[43]

"Interesting."

Puzzled that Jackson isn't making the connection, Jodi clarifies by saying, "My point is, as we age, like our parents, we may need help. That means our children get caught in the sandwich generation. Meaning we should probably look at what options are out there for us. I suggest a redo."

"A redo?"

"Of the three simple steps."

"Oh, yes, of course, I should have thought of that."

"We are in pretty good health, we are financially making good progress with our investments and savings, the kids are busy with their lives, and we are aware that extended health-care resources are not abundant. Why risk blowing up everyone's lifestyle and career paths if we can plan and take that risk off the table?"

"Let me set up a meeting to run this by the kids."

Now that everyone has been vaccinated, Jackson, Jodi, and Nicole get together at Erik's. Once they get the children settled for naps, Jackson opens up the conversation. Surprisingly, it's not that well received!

"First, I want to compliment both of you for how well you handled yourselves as part of your grandparents' Care Planning Team. They are adjusting to having help for Grandma, and you know Grandpa; he is controlling every detail of her care." Jackson pauses while his children brush off the compliment but beaming faces say otherwise.

Jodi puts her hand on Jackson's arm. "Now it's our turn."

Panic engulfs Erik's and Nicole's faces. They think they are about to hear that one of their parents has been diagnosed with something requiring extended care or worse.

Jodi continues, "Oh dear, I see I need to explain. One of our biggest concerns is that the obligation to provide extended or long-term care for one of us could likely interfere with your career path and your lifestyle." She can almost see behind their expressions that they are thinking about the promotion that she passed up and the terrible effect it had on her health. "Let me remind you that as we discovered workable options by using the three simple steps, the entire family, including your grandparents, started to look more relaxed and confident. We want to do the same for the next generation—you!"

Erik responds, "But isn't this too early? There isn't anything wrong, right?" Erik looks to his sister for backup.

Nicole takes over, "Is there something we don't know? I agree with Erik. Grandma and Grandpa are older. I am so glad that we found a couple of options that worked so they can age at home. But you guys are, well, younger."

Jodi answers, "As I recall, you both were concerned about the effect providing care for your grandparents was having on me, and that was before we ended up at the hospital. Erik, your job required you to move away. What if your or Nicole's next job or promotion moves you farther away? It is expensive to fly back and forth and not very practical."

Understandably, it is hard for Erik and Nicole to imagine their parents in need of extended or long-term care. So many images and activities on social media and advertising in general are geared toward remaining youthful. But that hasn't stopped the hands of time or events like the pandemic. Becoming a caregiver is not confined to just eldercare needs. Erik and Nicole gave Jackson a brochure to help Jodi realize that she and others were being negatively impacted by her caregiver duties. Now, it was her turn to share a chart.

Impact on Caregivers Finances, Work, and Lifestyle

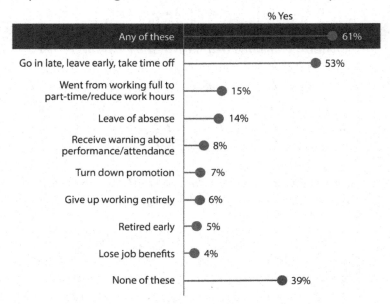

% Yes

Any of these	61%
Go in late, leave early, take time off	53%
Went from working full to part-time/reduce work hours	15%
Leave of absense	14%
Receive warning about performance/attendance	8%
Turn down promotion	7%
Give up working entirely	6%
Retired early	5%
Lose job benefits	4%
None of these	39%

"Caregiving in the US," Pew Research Center, Washington D.C. May 2020, Figure 69, accessed 12/05/2020
https://www.aarp.org/content/dam/aarp/ppi/2020/05/full-reort-caregiving-in-the-united-states.doi.10.26419-2F
ppi.00103.001.pdf

Jodi never indicated that caring for her parents had a financial impact on her retirement plans, although everyone suspected it went beyond the lost wages from passing on the promotion.

According to a Family Caregiving Cost survey, most family caregivers incur steep out-of-pocket costs related to caregiving. Long-distance caregivers, defined as family caregivers living more than one hour from the care recipient, incurred the highest out-of-pocket costs; however, even caregivers living with their care recipient incurred high costs.

The fact is, more than half of employed caregivers (56 percent) experience at least one work-related strain. It might mean working different hours, fewer or more hours, and taking time off, whether paid or unpaid. And then there is the effect on your own family if you need to cut back on other spending, which can undermine the family's future financial security. One in six caregivers in the survey reduced contributions to their retirement savings and roughly half have cut back on leisure spending."[44]

Jodi states her case. "Sixty-two percent of caregivers who participated in the AgingCare.com survey say that the cost of caring for a parent has impacted their ability to plan for their own financial future. This is simply not a risk that Dad and I are willing to take when at this age, we have other options."

Nicole, looking pensive, tries to wrap her head around why her parents are sharing this research, "So, what you're saying is that the age of a family member isn't the decisive factor but rather the serious consequences of not planning that you want to avoid, for all of us. What exactly are you suggesting?"

"Dad and I want to redo the three simple steps."

Erik, not aware of the potentially numerous available options, teases, "So, you and Dad intend to pay off your mortgage or maybe use Dad's veteran benefits?"

Jodi fakes an admonishing glance. "Since Dad and I are younger than Grandma and Grandpa and in relatively good health, there are many other options for us to consider."

"We know you would not hesitate to disrupt your lives and your careers to be our caregivers. And maybe you don't want to picture us seriously incapacitated due to an accident or illness or being at the same stage of care as your grandparents, but that just isn't realistic."

Jackson is more forceful in his approach. "We saw what caregiving did to Mom, and we simply do not want that for you. Here's what we will do. Let's arrange a series of Zoom calls since that worked pretty well before. Meanwhile, Mom and I will complete Step One and let you know our plans for Step Two."

Nicole looks hesitant. "OK, how many options are there? Maybe we could Zoom a little less frequently than we did with Grandma and Grandpa? We aren't as pressed, and I am struggling to see you needing care. Plus, I want to leave time in case I want to do additional research after we talk through potential options."

"In that case, why don't you set the schedule and send out calendar invites. We can deal with conflicts as we go. Meanwhile, have each of you put your Care Guide together?"

Erik quickly responds, "We did. We're almost done. We started with the children, and now we're doing ours. How about you, Nicole?"

Rolling her eyes at her brother, she replies, "Not yet. I'm busy! But I will get to it."

Playfully, Erik says, "Yup, looks like more work and investigation. Right up your alley, sis."

Takeaway:

Even after experiencing the demands and hardships associated with a family member's or friend's extended and long-term care, it is common to just put off planning for oneself. One of the unanticipated benefits of using the three simple steps is that CPT members, almost unconsciously, begin to internalize the possibilities and advantages of planning for themselves.

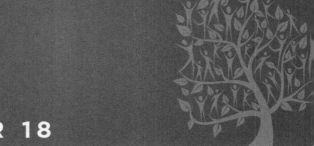

CHAPTER 18

Longevity and Retirement Create New Challenges

E rik and Nicole's reaction to planning for their parents is typical of their generation. It's a real struggle for younger generations to understand the positive role early long-term care planning plays in a secure lifestyle and retirement. But generations are living longer and longevity brings with it both the good and the less than good.

Volumes have been and continue to be written on the topic of longevity. Many people expect to depend on social security benefits to provide them with funds. Under current projections, the SSA Trustees say that reserves will be exhausted by the year 2034, after which time benefits may be reduced or, as in the past, Social Security taxes may be raised. That being said, even if retirement benefits are reduced, it's likely that the process will be gradual, and both current and future beneficiaries will be affected.

As we saw with the grandparents, when figuring social security benefits into your overall retirement or care needs financial picture, the trick is to understand some of the basic yet complex rules. And it is tricky! It is best to start with a simple grasp of foundational information. You can get a general sense of it by visiting the Social Security online services website.[45] There are also specialists and association websites [46] available to help you personalize and understand the impact of the various elections.

Another source of retirement income has seen major changes in the last decade.

The world of pension plans has dramatically changed over the years, moving away from defined benefit plans toward defined contribution plans. While a defined benefit plan provides a specified payment once you retire, a defined contribution plan is a savings plan that allows both employers (if they choose) and employees to contribute. The plan provides the employee with investment options. The plan also generally offers retiree payout options. Familiar examples of a defined contribution plan are 401(k) plans, 403(b) plans, employee stock ownership plans, and profit-sharing plans. A simplified employee pension (SEP) plan is a relatively uncomplicated retirement savings vehicle. These plans, properly invested, play an important role in retirement budgeting. Fortunately, both Jackson and Jodi have plans that will help secure their retirement unless they have unplanned extended and long-term care expenses.

The tendency is for the family to put off a redo for Jodi and Jackson even after sharing the sobering statistics of the impact that a lack of planning can have on retirement plans. Changing gears and bringing the discussion closer to home while having some fun by personalizing their longevity projections may do the trick. They will use a tool to estimate how many years they will need funds to support their retirement after leaving the workforce. The social security online estimator[47] shows the average number of additional years a person can expect to live, based only on the gender and date of birth you enter.

Jackson knew Erik's remark about more work was just teasing, but it gives him two ideas.

Jackson kicks off the Zoom call by saying, "Let's have some fun! I shared a link in the chat box for a site that allows us a peek at our expected longevity.

Nicole and Erik whip out their phones and start to play with the calculator.

After the kids have announced their expected projected longevity selves, and have sufficiently teased each other and their parents, Jackson gets their attention. "I'm glad you guys are enjoying this exercise. If you recall, while doing the three simple steps with your grandparents, we saw the impact of potential health-care costs on what your grandparents thought was a solid retirement income plan. You both have friends whose baby boomer parents or relatives have health issues or are experiencing the effects of aging."

Looking pensive, Nicole says, "True, we can relate. Our grandparents always seemed pretty healthy, but as they grew older, they needed more and more help. Since it was gradual, we sort of ignored it. Then the sudden emergency, and everything changed."

Sensitive to his mother's not sharing the impact it might have had on her finances, Erik ends the exchange on a positive note. "Under the emotional and financial cost umbrella, consequences might have spread far and wide. Creating that plan to include funding for long-term care expenses had a positive effect on their physical and emotional well-being."

Nicole gets her brother's drift. "And on all of us too!"

Jackson is pleased that the complaint about work has disappeared. He overreacted and was too sensitive. This little exercise was fun and made all of them think about the impact longevity can have on retirement and long-term care funding.

If it wasn't for sharing information about longevity and funding health-care costs during retirement, they probably would have underestimated the potential impact. And that's with Medicare deductibles and supplements at current pricing.

Jodi and Jackson, like so many workers, are in the prime earning years of their careers and are currently saving for retirement. But how many of us think about who is subsidizing our health-care costs? Currently, they participate in an employer-sponsored health-care plan. Costs are deducted directly out of their paycheck. It's easy to forget that during retirement, health-care costs are paid by the individual. Those are costs over which you have little control. They can rob you of the availability of retirement funds for other needs and activities. If chronic or serious long-term health issues arise, unplanned costs may further impact finances. Or what if you are young but surprised by an unplanned health event? Unfortunately, 37 percent of long-term care recipients are under sixty-five years old.[48]

Jackson circles back to how longevity could impact his and Jodi's retirement. "As we saw on the site, Mom's life expectancy means she will likely live a long time after she retires. If you think about it, you can control a certain amount of expenses in retirement, like housing costs, travel expenses, clothing, gifts, eating out, and accessory expenditures. Focusing on the long game, we will not have as much flexibility or control over health-care costs, such as Medicare or Medigap premiums, supplemental health insurance premiums, like vision or hearing, deductibles, copays, prescriptions, over-the-counter medicines, medical equipment, and support services and the wild card, extended or long-term care expenses.

After our experience with your grandparents, I started to read a good deal about retirement planning. According to a recent Edward Jones survey,[49] *'The new retirement is becoming an exciting and fulfilling stage of life—full of new choices, new freedoms, and new challenges.' Sounds great! Unless . . ."*

There is quite a bit of advertising in the news about retirement. You see much less on planning for future care needs. But as a recent Fox News article[50] noted, "The possibility of being able to enjoy and fund the lifestyle you want includes preparing for the possibility of needing care. Life insurance or long-term care insurance is also worth considering if you believe there's a chance you could one day require long-term care. [It] can exhaust even the largest emergency funds, so a long-term care policy or a life insurance policy with a long-term care rider can help you get the care you need without depleting your savings too quickly."

The key to avoid exhausting "even the largest emergency funds" is to plan in advance. The biggest advantage of advance planning is it opens up a pretty robust list of possible options for the CPT to consider.

"I think you now understand why a redo of the three simple steps for us is, well, simply smart. We don't want you to be caught in the sandwich generation. We will consider the impact of longevity on our retirement, especially on my side. We will carefully review how we figure in social security benefits and the availability of our pension funds and investment allocations. Neither of us wants to cause the other an unduly limited lifestyle by depleting our resources due to extended or long-term care needs.

And we have already gotten started. I am happy to report that Jackson and I have already completed Step One. We each created our own Care Guide. Next, we will lay out our Care Squad and get back to you. Stay well."

Takeaway:

Financial preparedness for living longer is more than a simple math problem. When leaving the workforce or retiring, remember that the costs for health care, health-care supplements, and extended and long-term care services are out of your control, making planning even more essential.

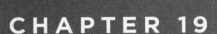

CHAPTER 19

Step Two:
Who Is Available in Person or
Virtually to Lend a Hand?

I f you recall, Jackson had two ideas. The first one involved making the homework more relatable for Erik and Nicole. The second one involved the formation of the Care Squad.

In the case of Jodi's parents, distance and availability was not a big issue. But that's not always the case.

No matter who you entrust with your Care Guide, relatives or even close friends may feel hurt or insulted at not being listed as the first line of help. You may need to explain why they are not the primary resource for the Care Squad.

Your primary responder should feel comfortable entering your house when you are not present. Additionally, you may want to let your local enforcement agency know your Care Squad person(s) is authorized to go into the empty home.

Another way to approach creating a Care Squad is to give a sealed copy of the Care Guide to the primary Care Squad person(s), who can then go straight to the hospital or care facility. You will need to remember to update the information.

We are getting to know the Jones family pretty well; let's see how they handle it.

> *After dinner, Jodi and Jackson, glass of wine in hand, move to the living room.*
>
> *Jackson doesn't turn the TV on.*
>
> *"What's up? You look as if you have something to tell me."*
>
> *"It's about forming the Care Squad. We probably should not have each other as the only primary person since we may be together. We still need to list Erik and Nicole but maybe we just give them a sealed copy so they don't have to go to the house before going to the hospital or care facility."*
>
> *"Good idea."*
>
> *"I'll let them know."*
>
> *After talking on the phone with Nicole, he turns back to Jodi. "Well, Nicole thought having a sealed copy made good sense."*
>
> *Jackson then calls Erik, hangs up, and looks at his wife.*
>
> *"What?"*
>
> *"Erik wants to have us put a copy in a sealed online vault. His friend owns a company that does just that.*

He will explain the security, access, and convenience to us. He said we should not be afraid to use technology. It does sound interesting."

Takeaway:

Technology advances provide, and will continue to provide, a boost to each of the three simple steps. Younger generations will look to available technologies to monitor care recipients, increase personal involvement, safely store documents, share information, and reduce reliance on face-to-face meetings, to name just a few.

CHAPTER 20

Step-Three: Expanding the Care Planning Team beyond Family

Although forming a Care Squad is a simple step, it must be practical and efficient in an emergency or over the long haul. For the CPT to be effective, it's much the same. All members must understand the basic objectives and rules. It isn't unusual to have more than just family members participate, but it should be clearly communicated why the Care Squad or CPT is expanding beyond the family. Nonfamily members need to understand their role in the Care Squad and the purpose, process, and promise of the CPT.

Jackson is lingering in the kitchen as Jodi makes a pot of coffee.

Jodi senses that there is something on Jackson's mind. She waits. Jackson seems hesitant.

"Let me guess. You want to have Doug as part of the Care Squad."

Jackson is stunned for a moment and then laughs. "Ah, well, yeah, I do."

"It' a great idea! Doug's over here a lot. He already has a spare key in case we lock ourselves out. Besides, Doug is the kind of friend that has become part of the family, if not by blood, then by his good heart, good sense, and loyalty."

Jackson volunteers to bring Doug up to speed on the Care Guide and his role as a primary responder for their Care Squad. Doug is flattered to be part of the Care Squad. But Jodi and Jackson want to take his involvement a step further.

"There is a third step in this planning process. Step Three of the three simple steps focuses on appropriate options to offset the risk of extended and long-term care. We would like you to be part of our Care Planning Team."

Doug, already impressed with the usefulness of Step One and the simplicity of Step Two, is curious about Step Three.

"Basically, Step Three is an education process. We take turns offering an overview of various extended and long-term care options. It will arm us with smart questions to ask a professional once we narrow down options to what we think works for us.

"I'm in!"

In general, and in particular for creating a group such as the CPT, to work effectively together, clear and open communication channels are essential. Your CPT may span several generations, making tolerance and recognition of generational orientations critical components.

Jackson, Jodi, and Doug are part of the baby boomer generation, born between 1946 and 1964. As we often hear, the baby boomer generation is an extremely large cohort in part due to the relative political stability after the Second World War. As a generation, they tend to be much more optimistic than their parents, the silents, due to the economic boom from postwar reconstruction and the following years of steady industrial development. Many baby boomers tended to reject the traditional values of their parents, and they became much more individualistic and liberal. Many idealistically looked for social change and experimented with different ideas, lifestyles, sexual freedoms, and ways of thinking.

Understanding members of the CPT in terms of their personal and lifestyle influencers can involve research or simply sharing memories.

Let's continue as Jackson and Doug stroll down memory lane.

"Do you remember the hippie movement during the late sixties?"

Taking a drink of his beer, Jackson looks nostalgic as he replies, "Yes, so many of our boomer friends were free-spirited, open, and interested in social causes. We saw the civil rights, antiwar, and women's movements emerge, and politics become a mass event where I think two more or less defined sides—liberalism and conservatism—became more evident."

"The kids think we are relics when it comes to technology, but we witnessed the rapid development of technology, came to appreciate it, and accepted it. I remember hearing the terms space race *and* arms race, *we saw the*

invention of the transistor and the television, and we lived through the Green Revolution in agriculture."

"Which the kids now consider old school. They even watch their programs on their phones!"

Undeterred, Jackson presses on. "And don't forget the great advances in medicine. Remember how crazy and almost scary it was when they did the first heart transplant? Nowadays, they transplant all sorts of—"

Jodi enters the room and interjects, chuckling, "Parts!"

They share a laugh and Doug wraps up. "Then, when some of our baby boomer friends got to the top of the corporate and political ladders, their conservatism became evident. The words politically correct *became a euphemism for taboo subjects."*

The friends are enjoying their shared memories, but they will have to keep in mind that their children come with very different life experiences and are grown adults. They were willing to take a back seat while participating in planning for their grandparents, but when it comes to their own parents, it's closer to home. It can be a different story.

Erik is part of Generation X, born within the years 1965–1980. Growing up during the final years of the Vietnam War, Watergate, and the Reagan and Bush Senior era, GenXers witnessed the end of the Cold War, the expansion of globalism, the introduction of early home computers, radical changes to the media industry, and the early days of MTV. They grew up with continual change and the introduction of new technologies. Thus, they are accustomed to a changing environment. [51]

Nicole is a member of the millennial generation, born between the years 1981–1996. They grew up with continual advancements in technology. They are comfortable accessing online retail and sharing all sorts of opinions and information. They exhibit a discernable preference for experiences over products. They research before they commit. They have brought racial and ethnic diversity to the forefront of American society. And millennial women, like Generation X women, are more likely to participate in the nation's workforce than prior generations. Compared with previous generations, millennials—the oldest one turned forty in 2021—are delaying or foregoing marriage and have been somewhat slower in forming their own households. [52]

As the mother of both a GenXer who came into the workforce on the cusp of cell phones, the Internet, and social media, and the mother of a millennial, who grew up when these things were a regular part of daily life, Jodi is aware that her children's approach to using the three simple steps may vary from hers. She is concerned that Jackson will not appreciate that the children were generationally distanced from planning for their grandparents but this time, it's much closer to home for them.

Back at the Jones house, the doorbell rings. Jackson ushers Doug in and hands him a cold beer.

"Thanks for coming." Turning toward the kitchen, he shouts, "Honey, Doug is here, so let's get started."

Jodi is glad to see Doug and really pleased to have him as a member of the CPT. Doug will be less sensitive about certain issues than her husband (and maybe herself as well). "We completed Step One, and you now know where we keep our Care Guides. You have our completed Step Two Care Squad chart. Now onto Step Three."

"I explained to Doug," evidently, Jackson expects to take the lead, "that our goal is to effectively reduce a whole bunch of negative consequences resulting from not being prepared for extended or long-term care. 'Plan for the unplanned' is the way I put it. I already discussed with

Doug how effective it was to have multiple generations on board for when what we thought might eventually happen with your parents, suddenly did!"

"Yes, it could have been a real nightmare, but we all handled it pretty well."

Jackson's tone softens as he describes how on a very personal level, having a plan for Jodi's parents also avoided interfering with continuing their contributions to 401k plans, investments, and the 529 plans they set up for funding their grandchildren's education.

Clearly impressed, Doug asks, "And you're sure the kids are OK with my being part of this?"

"Oh yeah, Erik told me that you probably remember my personal and family history better than I do!"

The look exchanged between Jodi and Doug says that there is probably some truth to that statement.

The Jones are ready to kick off their CPT meetings. Jodi volunteers to be the secretary. When working with a larger CPT, it is helpful to send a brief summary of each call to each of the members. It keeps everyone on the same page and serves as a reminder of progress being made. In the future, if emotions run high, it will help to remind everyone how and why decisions were made.

Takeaway:

Whether a close friend or trusted advisor, having an unrelated person as part of your CPT can be very helpful since they are less emotionally invested in every issue and may offer other avenues to explore.

CHAPTER 21

Envisioning Your Future Self through Self-Profiling

T he nicest thing about the future is that it always starts tomorrow. Speaking of the future, one of the hardest things about planning for the future is imagining what it will bring. In the case of extended or long-term care planning, a helpful technique is to imagine that an extended care plan you envision has succeeded. From that point, think through all the reasons why it would be successful. Then, imagine that the same strategy has underperformed, and think through all the reasons why it wouldn't achieve success.

For someone struggling to envision their future self, here are some helpful questions to help guide you. Each person should answer them individually.

- Do you have a retirement date in mind?
- If applicable, do you think your spouse/partner has the same date in mind?

- Will you want to travel? Do you have a budget for travel and entertainment in mind?
- Do you expect to do volunteer work?
- How do you envision your health during the aging process?
- Do you expect to stay in your current home and age in place, downsize, or change homes?
- Do you want to stay in your current location or move closer to your children or friends?
- Do you want to live independently if your spouse/partner/ companion predeceases you?
- Do you worry about affording the lifestyle you envision?
- Do you worry about being a burden?
- What do you want to leave behind as a legacy?
- Do you have a story about someone close in age to you who had extended or long-term care needs? What happened? Does their story affect your view? Do you think their story adds color to how you envision your story?

Jackson and Jodi found the exercise personally helpful, enlightening, and fun!

"I wish I had been a fly on the wall," Doug jokes. " Did you two do serious battle?"

"There is no denying that at times, it got, shall we say, a bit informative. But it's what you don't know that you don't know that can trip you up."

"Or what you think you know that you don't know," Doug observes.

"At the end of the day, or shall I say, at the end of multiple dinners, we had a much better idea of why people turn to advisors for help," Jackson hesitantly admits.

"You mean as a referee?"

Jackson, now grinning, replies, " I guess!" Then, more seriously, he adds, "But more as an interpreter to help us see possibilities."

Although Jodi and Jackson may have envisioned things differently, they probably heard an occasional response from each other that helped broaden their perspective. To further boil it down to what is essential, each person should write down five or six key words to describe how they envision a future care needs plan as a way to conclude the exercise. It is important to remember that it is not about a process, not about a product, not yet about a plan, but about you.

As a result of the exercise, on the next CPT call, Jodi shares the chart that she and Jackson put together. "This is a quick summary of what we have gathered from documentation, planning exercises, and conversations."

J&J Boomer Summary

	Jackson	Jodi
Health	Good	Preferred
Family health history	Average	Longevity
Wealth category	Middle income family	Middle income family
Location - current	Madison, WI	Madison, WI
Location - future	Unsure	Wisconsin Dells
Role of current insurances	Possible 1035 exchange	Possible term conversion
Funding for 1035 exchange or replacement of current insurance policy	From current life policy group life policy	Possible term replacement
Savings	401K HSA	401K HSA
Liquid assets	Joint savings account	Joint savings account
Desired location if extended or long term care are needed	Assisted Living Facility	Assisted Living Facility or Continuing Care Retirement Community
Family/friends/government serve as caregivers	Yes	No
Retirement	Age 70	Age 65-67
Couples potential caregiving responsibilities	Yes parents / yes children	No parents / yes children

As the CPT reviews the chart, Jodi makes additional comments.

- *Jackson and I have a mortgage on our home that we are not planning to pay off.*
- *We usually rent that lake cottage near Jackson's parents during our vacation and attend Jackson's annual family reunion. We love it there and would consider spending part of the year there. Maybe we'll even retire there since it is a familiar and affordable area. And Jackson's parents would like us to live close to them. We have a friend who has moved into an assisted living facility in that area and seems quite satisfied with the arrangement.*
- *We both participate in our employers' qualified savings plans, which are 401(k) plans. Both employers offer contributions for participants—at least they did pre-COVID.*
- *We sometimes carry a small running debt on our credit cards.*
- *We access health-care coverage through Jackson's employment.*
- *We both have group disability insurance. Jackson has an additional disability insurance policy that he carries due to the home mortgage.*
- *We both contribute to individual health savings accounts.*
- *I envision retiring before Jackson, who wants to collect the optimal amount of social security benefits for which he can qualify since currently there is a financial bonus for delayed retirement.*

Nicole and Erik simultaneously ask, "What kind of financial bonus?"

New Tools to Review Social Security Benefits

One thing that comes up during the future self-exercise is that people have different ideas about when they want to retire and when to collect social security benefits. As we previously saw, the grandparents' assessment of Social Security income and the ongoing support it may or may not provide differs from Jackson's expectations.

Generally speaking, a delay in claiming benefits results in receiving a monthly benefit that is 8 percent higher for each year a person puts off collecting benefits. If your full retirement age (FRA) is sixty-seven years but you postpone claiming benefits until age seventy, the benefit—at least currently—will be 24 percent higher. But that 8 percent increase doesn't account for the fact that Jackson will miss out on three full years' worth of Social Security checks. Jackson should dig deeper to really understand how he may or may not benefit from delaying collecting benefits, just as Jodi should understand the rules for collecting benefits before her FRA.

Aside from consulting a social security specialist, the Social Security Administration offers a helpful website.[53] In May 2021, the Social Security Administration rolled out a new Social Security statement. Once you create your My Social Security account[54], the website offers one of the most telling and effective tools a person can use to learn about their earnings and future social security benefits. Rather than providing information for just ages sixty-two, sixty-seven, and seventy, the new format shows what the estimated monthly benefits would be for each year if you start receiving benefits anytime within the ages of sixty-two and seventy. The information is shown as a personalized graphic with a series of horizontal bars.

When you access your statement in your My Social Security account, there are links to nine online supplemental fact sheets.

Jackson concludes, "It appears that a wise direction would be to include social security benefits in an envisioned proposed plan but not rely solely on them as a major source of income for funding care."

Nicole picks up the conversation, adding, "During the planning session with my grandparents, we saw the potentially serious financial impact of relying on social security income if one of them predeceases the other."

Doug responds, as if on cue, "Funny you mention that, Nicole. My oldest sister is living with her husband in a CCRC, which is a continuing care retirement community. The family continually teases her about taking such good care of him. Aside from the fact that they have been together for a very long time, the truth is she worries that either one of them may not be able to afford the cost of living in the CCRC if his or her social security income or a portion of their pension income is eliminated. The CCRC maintenance costs are adjusted for inflation each year. She doesn't feel she has much wiggle room. We all tease her about keeping him alive!"

"Jodi, why don't we continue with the summary," Jackson suggests, feeling the point is made and hopefully absorbed.

"Right" Jodi refocuses, "Once we finish the summary, we can start to consider the extended and long-term care options available to us."

Jodi continues with the summary:

- *Jackson has a whole life insurance policy that he bought years ago. Jackson qualifies for his employer's group life policy for two times his salary.*

- *I have a term life insurance policy. I don't have additional life insurance coverage through my workplace.*
- *We have a joint investment account from which we recently withdrew a small amount in order to help Erik and his wife pay bills for a complicated health issue that their son experienced.*
- *Jackson is a very proud veteran. He and Doug served together.*
- *We completed health and property directives, DNR paperwork, and so on. We also created a living will."*
- *I am willing to consider moving into an assisted living facility or CCRC but only if it provides a continuum for more extensive care in case one or both of us experience serious health issues.*

The question of where you will live in retirement should not be overlooked in the planning process. The grandparents planned to age in their home and paid off their mortgage with that goal in mind. Jodi and Jackson may consider an alternate living arrangement. While some assisted living facilities (ALF) have added services and are run more like a CCRC, ALFs are licensed to deal mostly with those who are impaired. Some independent living facilities are adding services, incorporating them as ALFs too. There are important differences in these options, so a close look at details based on your personal expectations is a wise use of planning time.

Takeaway:

It is challenging to objectively fast-forward our future self and especially challenging to envision future care settings, costs, and funding. Using available tools and paying attention to differences and similarities between partners will pay off!

CHAPTER 22

Moving Your Extended or Long-Term Care Plan Forward

The Care Planning Team is sharing stories, envisioning future plans, and employing longevity and cost of care tools while reviewing Jodi and Jackson's summary. Let's see what else moves the decision-making process along.

"Hi, everyone, one of the great side effects of being a part of the Care Planning Team (CPT) is that we all get together on a regular schedule. I think we are all benefiting from this learning process. Let's have some fun. This guessing game relates to possible retirement locations and their various care costs. Who would like to guess as to how many counties there are in the United States?"

Each CPT member throws out a number.

"Doug guessed 2,850 and that was the closest. Currently, there are 3,006 counties in the United States alongside 142 county-equivalents, like boroughs in Alaska and parishes in Louisiana.[55] Keep in mind that costs and local services may vary from one area to another.

"What's my prize?" Doug asks.

"You don't wind up receiving care at a location that isn't your first choice!"

"Good point! By taking the current monthly cost and then using one of the insurance geographical cost-of-care calculators[56] to push it out twenty-five years, I can estimate how much money I would have to save to cover costs in various settings and locations."

Nicole does some quick math. "Wow! The aging baby boomer population is estimated to be about 72 million people. It's impossible to know where costs will go, other than up! Let's just confidently conclude that it is likely to be a significant number."

"Even if I gave up my favorite restaurant, wine, and poker games, "Jackson says, grinning at Doug, "I don't see us saving that kind of money!"

Jodi nods and says, "Or keeping that amount of money in an emergency fund earning next to nothing! Bottom line, Dad and I don't want to be obligated to keep that amount of money in a low-risk investment, designated only as an emergency extended or long-term care fund. We want to leverage our money by insuring against funding those ever-increasing costs. More importantly, we

*want to do it while we qualify for several options so we
have choices."*

*Doug is starting to clearly see the reason his friends want
to plan now. "Even with a good financial plan in place,
I guess someone who doesn't plan for possible extended or
long-term care costs may be obligated to withdraw savings, cash in stocks, or liquidate assets regardless of good
or bad market timing. I wonder what our tax advisor
would say."*

*Jackson, who uses the same CPA as Doug, remarks,
"Nothing that I would want to hear!"*

Having your savings and accumulated assets blow up probably
wouldn't make for a pretty tax picture. It leaves you vulnerable and
dependent on family and friends, or government, state, and/or community services. Expecting help from outside resources comes with
emotional complications for both the giver and the receiver. It can
mean that someone else or an entity may control your care. That's an
unsettling prospect.

Looking into funding vehicles early in your career while there
is ample time to accumulate funds is smart. One way to contribute
funds to retirement income is with a Health Savings Account (HSA).
An HSA is specifically designed to help pay for medical care costs and,
under certain circumstances, long-term care insurance premiums.
According to their personal summary, Jodi and Jackson both have
HSA accounts.

Takeaway:

Paying for extended or long-term care expenses is an income problem that can have serious asset, investment, and personal preference
consequences.

CHAPTER 23

A Health Savings Account as a Funding Mechanism

A health savings account (HSA) is a tax-advantaged medical savings account that allows account holders to save money for the payment of health-care costs for themselves and their families. HSA funds roll over from year to year with no use-it-or-lose-it limits and can be invested like a 401(k). The contributions are either pretax or tax-deductible. The interest and earnings in an HSA grow tax free and withdrawals for qualified medical expenses are also tax free.

You can use your HSA funds to pay for your spouse or tax dependents' qualified medical expenses tax free, even if they're on different health plans or ineligible to contribute to HSAs. There is a helpful website that lists qualified medical expenses, such as doctor's visits, prescriptions, dental bills, and more.[57]

If you become ineligible to contribute to your HSA, you can continue to pay for qualified medical expenses tax free from the funds currently in your account. Health savings account regulations are being updated to keep up with current advances in care. Due to COVID-19, the Coronavirus Aid, Relief, and Economic Security Act (CARES ACT) [58] made some significant changes. One such change permitted the use of savings to include coverage for telehealth services. We'll have to see if it becomes permanent.

If you contribute to your HSA via pretax payroll withholding through your employer's Section 125 plan, you don't pay FICA taxes on those contributions.[59] Because HSAs are individually owned, they stay with you when you change jobs or retire.

You can use HSA funds tax free to pay for qualified long-term care insurance premiums.[60] The maximum annual tax-free amount is based on your age. The age-based limit modestly increases each year.

HSAs are not only tax-advantaged savings accounts, but individual account holders may invest the funds. You may choose one or both of these investment options: an interest-bearing investment account or an interest-bearing debit account. As part of your protection plan, they help avoid depleting a comprehensive retirement package by helping to pay for long-term care insurance premiums and medical expenses.

Jodi and Jackson mention health savings plans to the CPT as a future payment method if they purchase an insurance product. "Did you know that you can use an HSA account as a long-term care funding mechanism?"

Everyone shakes their heads. "Don't feel bad. We also thought you couldn't use an HSA account to pay for long-term care premiums, and we actually have HSAs! It's a popular misconception when it comes to paying long-term care premiums. Although HSA funds cannot be used to pay regular health insurance premiums, Dad and I can withdraw money from either or both of our HSAs to pay for specialized types of insurance, such as long-term care insurance."

Erik, looking hopeful, asks, "I have a flexible savings account at work? Is that the same?"

"No, sorry dear, it isn't. But I am glad you asked. It's easy to mix the two up since both FSAs and HSAs are pretax accounts you can use to pay for health-care related expenses."

It is not uncommon to be confused about FSA versus HSA accounts.

- Both flexible savings accounts (FSA) and health savings accounts offer tax benefits.
- Both accounts have annual contribution limits.[61]
- FSAs can work like a line of credit. You can use your FSA to cover eligible health-care expenses early in the year. Let's say you need a $300 pair of glasses but you only have $200 currently saved in the FSA. As long as your plan allows and you plan to contribute $300 to the FSA by the end of the year, you can purchase the glasses when you need them. On the other hand, HSA holders can't spend more than the funds that have been deducted from their paycheck or funds they have contributed to an HSA at a bank or other institution. Otherwise, you would have to file for a deduction later in the year.
- You cannot contribute to an HSA and a traditional FSA in the same year.
- FSAs work on a use-it-or-lose-it basis. If you don't spend the funds by the end of the plan year, you lose them unless your employer's plan offers a grace period or a rollover period (or, as was the case during the COVID-19 pandemic, the regulation is altered or suspended).
- HSA accounts may offer investment options.
- And importantly, only HSAs (as opposed to FSAs) can be used to pay long-term care premiums.

Let's see how the CPT reacts to this long-term care funding option.

Having piqued everyone's interest, Jodi throws out a second question. "How would anyone who is not contributing to an FSA account open an HSA account?"

"You better just tell us, Mom." Nicole is ready for more details.

Jodi explains, "Actually, there are two ways to open an HSA account. Since the HSA belongs to the individual and not the employer, as long as you are covered by a high deductible health plan, or HDHP, you may open and contribute to an HSA. The other way is how Dad and I did it. Since we have a qualifying HDHP through work, we were also able to open an HSA through our employer."

Nicole continues her inquiry. "What if my employer doesn't offer an HSA account? Where can I open one on my own?"[62]

Jodi answers, "First, remember that you cannot contribute to both an HSA and FSA. From what I read, Nicole, you may want to check first with your human resources department since my employer, like others, contributes money to my HSA. I suspect that my employer may pick up the fees as well. If that's not an option, when I was reading about funding a long-term care policy with HSA funds, I came across an online search site to help you find an HSA administrator.[63]

You can compare fees and investing options. I'm sure there are other such sites as well."

"For what it's worth, let me pitch in here." All eyes shift to Doug. "I opened an HSA account at my company, and I have my contribution deducted from my pay. Since I contribute to my HSA via pretax payroll withholding through my employer's Section 125 plan, I don't pay FICA taxes on those contributions. Currently, that means an extra 7.65 percent from each contribution comes back to me.[64] And because HSAs are individually owned, it will stay with me if I change jobs or retire." Clearing his throat, Doug continues, "Let me read you the information I have from when I signed up for my HSA at work. We were told that you can use an HSA account for tax-free withdrawals to pay a portion of long-term care insurance premiums with limitations based on your age. After you turn sixty-five, you can use HSA money to pay premiums for Medicare Part A, B, or D as well as qualified copays for Part D. Medicare Advantage, Medicare HMO, and MAPD plan premiums are also eligible expenses for reimbursement as well as long-term care insurance premiums.

You must consult with your tax advisor, but let's discuss the deductibility of qualified premium payments. After retirement, income tends to drop and medical, dental, vision, and hearing expenses often increase. Adding a tax-qualified long-term care insurance (LTCI) premium payment may help you qualify for the federal tax deduction. Surprisingly, the rules are pretty straightforward and differences between the federal tax deduction and HSA tax deduction surface.

- Federal tax deduction (under IRC §7702B and IRC §213)
  - Currently, you must meet a 10% floor of Adjusted Gross Income (AGI) in out-of-pocket medical expenses
    o If someone's AGI equals $100,000,

    o   then, $10,000 must be paid out of pocket before any deduction applies.

    o   Deductions are limited to IRS age-based deduction limits.

- HSA deduction
  - No 10 percent floor to meet
  - Deduction limited to IRS age-based distribution limits
  - You'll owe taxes on non-health-care withdrawals after 65, but in that case the HSA is receiving the same tax treatment as a tax-sheltered account as an IRA or 401(k).

Nicole is the detail person in the CPT. Although the CPT is concentrating on options for her parents, she shares her thoughts about establishing an HSA for the future funding of a qualified policy. "I see the advantages for Erik of contributing to an FSA given his young family, but as a single person, I want to look at this option more closely for myself as a potential future funding option.

Let's say I open an HSA. Let's also assume that over the years I want to maximize my annual contributions. I access the IRS website and respect the updated annual limits for HSA contributions as well as the minimum deductible and maximum out-of-pocket expenses for the HDHPs with which the HSAs are paired. Then, let's also assume I am eligible to take an HSA distribution for my LTCI premiums. It will be the lesser of premiums paid or age-based limits. If that's my plan, the long-term care insurance policy I purchase must be a qualified long-term care insurance contract. If I consider a hybrid or linked policy, I will ask to see the information in writing or an illustration provided by the insurer indicating any portion of the policy that meets the criteria to make some of the paid premium eligible toward tax deductibility thresholds. Sounds like it could be a good direction for me to go!"

HSA Accounts

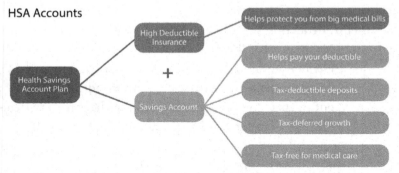

Because the administration of an HSA is a taxpayer responsibility, advisors and consumers are strongly encouraged to consult a tax advisor before opening an HSA. Information is available from the Internal Revenue Service (IRS) for taxpayers, which can be found online at the IRS website at IRS.gov IRS Publication 969, Health Savings Accounts and Other Tax-Favored Health Plans, and IRS Publication 502, Medical and Dental Expenses, online, by calling the IRS to request a copy of each at 800.829.3676

Takeaway:

No matter what age, how, or when it fits into your budget or plan for medical care needs, HSAs offer triple tax advantages. Funded HSAs provide a good option for paying future long-term care premium payments.

CHAPTER 24

What Are the Options for the Healthy and Not So Healthy?

S o far, the Jones family CPT has reviewed four funding options:

- They examined the advantages of using HSA account money to help fund insurance policy premium payments.
- They reviewed the reliability of depending on social security benefits as a major source of income for funding care.
- They considered the desirability of segmenting a large sum of funds for the payment of long-term care expenses.
- They realized the instability of relying on invested funds for payments, which could lead to unfortunate market timing and tax implications.

Having eliminated those options, the CPT continues to look at the range of options with the objective of ensuring their personal preferences are met without destroying lifestyles or family ties.

For someone in good or relatively good health, insurance options include the following:

- Traditional long-term care (TLTC)
- Worksite group long-term care (GLTC)
- Whole and universal life insurance
- Life insurance with riders
- Annuities with riders
- Term insurance with riders

For someone with some health issues or budget concerns, insurance and noninsurance options include the following:

- Short-term care
- Reverse mortgage
- Life settlements

For impaired health cases, insurance and noninsurance options include the following:

- Single premium immediate annuities (SPIA)
- Veterans benefits
- Medicare (benefits are limited)

For someone who meets the definition of impoverished, noninsurance options include the following:

- Medicaid
- State and county services

"Wow, I am surprised by the number of options available to you guys." Erik's expression reveals that he is both surprised and pleased. "Now I see why you insisted on

moving forward with the three simple steps. Compared to my grandparents, this is a whole different scenario."

Jodi replies, "True! Our advisor is a member of a professional association called the National Association of Insurance and Financial Advisors, or NAIFA. It provides her with access to specialists who sponsor the NAIFA Limited and Extended Care Planning Center.[65] Additionally, NAIFA has extensive partners and works closely with other associations, which expands her ability to access additional resources. After we became more familiar with what Grandpa agreed was a workable option, she introduced us to specialists who helped us dig into the details of both government programs and some noninsurance options for my parents. With the help of that team, we quickly and successfully arranged a funded plan that works for them."

"What she suggests for this CPT is not an in-depth analysis but a basic overview of options." Smiling, she adds, "We don't want to become paralyzed by information overload; we just want to become educated consumers"

Jackson, who sees this exercise as beneficial for all adds, "And learning isn't just for mom's and my benefit. Once you expand your knowledge base, when you do meet with an advisor or agent, you can explain the direction you may want to go, or at least ask good questions."

Nicole smiles. "Perfect!"

Becoming familiar with options in order to effectively plan is a "perfect" step, but there is no such thing as a perfect solution. Underwriting, product availability, state requirements, cost, and riders (add-on benefits or options, company ratings, etc.) may impact the selection. In addition, postponing or not moving ahead with a plan may result in you being ineligible for a plan option that would have fit your needs and budget if you had acted earlier.

There is a popular saying in the long-term care insurance business: Your health buys you insurance; your money just pays for it.

Jodi and James make a list of insurance options they want to consider while they are still eligible. The CPT members choose various insurance options to examine.

A Brief History of Long-Term Care Insurance

Before looking at insurance options, it is helpful to understand some insurance basics. According to Wikipedia, insurance is a contract, represented by a policy, in which an individual or entity receives financial protection or reimbursement against losses. The company pools clients' risks to make payments more affordable for the insured.

LTC insurance was first offered to US consumers in 1974. At the time, LTC insurance had no targeted regulatory guidance or consumer protections in place. Recognizing the need, the National Association of Insurance Commissioners (NAIC) released the Long-Term Care Insurance Model Act (1987) and Long-Term Care Insurance Model Regulation (1988) to provide state regulators with a set of minimum standards and practices. Over the years, the NAIC have adopted additional standards. While state regulations ultimately govern the LTC insurance product, federal regulations have influenced the product structure and state adoption of NAIC standards.[66]

By the 1980s, long-term care insurance was becoming popular.[67] Due to advances in medicine and science, life expectancy was steadily increasing, with more consumers becoming aware of the need to fund potential long-term care needs. Insurers responded by creating additional products. By the 1990s, LTC insurance was regularly being sold.

On August 21, 1996, President Bill Clinton signed the Health Insurance Portability and Accountability Act (HIPAA) into law. The release of HIPAA, and its associated updates, have provided provisions that offer tax-qualified status to policies that comply with certain criteria, such as offering inflation protection and utilizing disability status as a benefit trigger.[68]

HIPAA states that LTC insurance will be treated in the same manner as health and accident insurance under the Federal Income Tax Code. This means that benefits paid by a policy will not be counted as taxable income to the policyholder.

Under HIPAA, benefit triggers are defined and used to determine when a policyholder is considered chronically ill and thus eligible to claim for benefits. A licensed health-care practitioner must certify that the insured;

- has a severe cognitive impairment that requires continual supervision to prevent them from harming themselves or others and
- is unable to perform without "substantial assistance" from another individual at least two activities of daily living (ADL) for a period of at least 90 days due to a loss of functional capacity. The activities of daily living are bathing, continence, dressing, eating, toileting, and transferring (e.g., getting out of a bed and into a chair).

In the late 1980s, the Robert Wood Johnson Foundation supported the development of a new LTC insurance model, with the goal of encouraging more people to purchase LTC coverage. The RWJ Partnership program, commonly called the Partnership for Long-Term Care,[69] brought states and private insurers together to create a new insurance product aimed at moderate-income individuals or those at most risk of future reliance on Medicaid to cover long-term care needs. States offer the guarantee that if benefits under a Partnership policy do not sufficiently cover the cost of care, the consumer may qualify for

Medicaid under special eligibility rules while retaining a prespecified amount of assets (income and functional Medicaid eligibility rules still apply). Thus, the consumer is protected from having to become impoverished to qualify for Medicaid. Four states—California, Connecticut, Indiana, and New York—implemented Partnership programs in the early 1990s. However, the Omnibus Budget Reconciliation Act (OBRA) of 1993 enacted restrictions on the further development of these type of state partnership programs. The four states with existing Partnership programs were allowed to continue. Indiana, however, is working through the details of moving from a RWJ Partnership to a DRA Partnership program.

In 2005, the Deficit Reduction Act (DRA),[70] authorized states (outside of the original four RWJ states) to offer special Medicaid asset disregards for people purchasing and using qualified private long-term care insurance policies. Popularly referred to as Partnership Policies, the program allows individuals to protect some or all of their assets and still qualify for Medicaid if their long-term care needs extend beyond the period covered by their private insurance policy. The DRA requires programs to include certain consumer protections; in addition, policies must include inflation protection when purchased by a person under age seventy-six.[71]

As the LTC marketplace evolves, insurers and marketers enter and exit the market at various times for different reasons. Options for long-term and extended care needs have evolved and will continue to evolve. As we will see during the overview of multiple insurance options, HIPAA does *not* apply to all long-term care insurance policies that use riders to cover LTC risk. HIPAA's provisions only apply to what it defines as tax-qualified long-term care insurance contracts. A tax-qualified LTCI contract meets federal standards and offers tax advantages to the buyer.

No matter which products the CPT looks at, they will ultimately want to review each option with an advisor, agent, specialist, or tax consultant in terms of the following:

- What does it do?
- What does it *not* do?
- What is the premium payment schedule?
- What happens if you miss a payment?
- What are the basic benefits?
- What benefit riders are available, and what is the effect of adding benefit riders?
- How much money does the policy provide for services and funding?
- When does it provide for services and funding? What are the benefit triggers?
- What method is used to compensate you for services received?
- How long does it provide for those services and funding?
- Are there any tax implications you should be aware of?

Takeaway:

Over a relatively short period of time, numerous extended and long-term care options have developed and are continuing to develop and evolve to serve many different health and financial circumstances. There is a right one for you if you take the time to really understand your potential needs, ask the right questions, and plan.

CHAPTER 25

The Pros and Cons of Traditional Long-Term Care

Understanding the history of LTC insurance helps the CPT understand how young the LTC industry is compared to other types of insurance. After all, modern insurance can be traced back to the Great Fire of London of 1666. The first American insurance company was organized by Ben Franklin in 1752, and the first life insurance company was organized in 1759. We can expect additional limited, extended, and long-term care options to emerge.

Jodi is somewhat familiar with the first option, TLTC, since she called out some facts that removed it from consideration for her parents. Since she and Jackson are younger and in better health, it may be a viable option for either or both of them.

"I mentioned this option during my parent's CPT, but Jackson and I are in better health, we are younger, and

our finances are still growing—so it's a very different scenario.

Traditional long-term care (TLTC) insurance may also be referred to as stand-alone LTC. Some advisors refer to it as pure protection since unlike some other insurance options where policies combine different coverages, TLTC focuses solely on offsetting expenses for a long-term care need. TLTC policies are underwritten for morbidity not mortality."

"Mom, we better have whoever is presenting define words the way insurance companies define or use them," *says Nicole.*

Nicole reminds us of a very important point. As you review products, it is very important to understand insurance lingo. Words have different connotations depending on the context in which they are used. Know the definitions of key words in the context of an insurance policy so you and the insurer are on the same page.

For example, *morbidity* is not just feeling gloomy or morbid, which is how most of us define the word. In insurance lingo, morbidity refers to having a disease or a symptom of a disease.

Examples of morbidity include injuries from motor vehicle accidents, drug poisoning, falls, or violence; other examples include infectious diseases like the COVID-19 virus, other influenzas, foodborne illness, health care-associated infections, and sexually transmitted infections.

Mortality refers to the state of being mortal or destined to die. In medicine and long-term care insurance, the term is also used for death rate, or the number of deaths in a certain group of people during a certain period of time.

The CPT adopts the policy of clarifying words using the specific definition employed by the insurance product as one of its rules.

Jodi continues, "Understandably, someone suffering from a morbid illness or disease when they apply for TLTC will be charged more than someone in good health since logically they are probably closer to claiming benefits than someone in better health.

Many consumers and advisors still consider TLTC a solid option because TLTC policies typically offer more comprehensive coverage since they are solely focused on offsetting the extended or long-term care risk. Plus, there is usually a good deal of benefit design flexibility."

Erik observes, "Sounds like TLTC could be the foundation for a good extended or long-term care plan. I think I hear a 'but' coming, Mom. So is there an issue?"

Jodi's son brings up another important element of an overview; pair the good with the not-so-good issues that may be attached to a product. In the case of TLTC, unfortunately, older policies have incurred the ire of the press and the public due to increased premium payments. Additionally, older negative statistical marketing led many people to immediately associate long-term care with diminished health and loss of independence. Due to negative stories in the press, rarely mentioning the *billions* that the industry has paid out in claims, many people associate long-term care with nursing home insurance or rate increases.

Other CPT members share firsthand experiences that resonate and contribute to the learning process.

Doug adds, "One of my buddy's parents had rate increases on their policy. They weren't at all happy!"

"What did they do about it?" Nicole asks.

"They said that the insurance company included alternate premium payment offers in the letter they received about the rate increase. Their agent also received a copy of the letter containing various alternate premium payment options. They reviewed and discussed the alternate offers together. They opted for one that fit their current situation so they were comfortable keeping the policy. Besides, when they looked at the cost of a current policy or other coverages, it made the increased premium seem pretty decent for the coverage!"

While receiving a rate increase is not great news, a brief look at TLTC rate increase history offers some insight. Pricing for early products was based on historical behavior of the owners of other insurances, such as life insurance. The reason for increased premiums is not a simple calculation. When requesting a rate increase, the insurer is obligated to make a sound financial case to each state where that policy was sold. The state may grant the premium increase request or modify it before granting the request. The need for additional carrier profit is not a valid argument.

Hindsight is a powerful educator. Actuaries now have a couple of decades of history to examine. Pricing is now more conservative because interest rates are, and have been for some time, at historical lows, lapse rates (the expectation that people will cancel their policies or die before claiming benefits) have been effectively de-risked, and both mortality and morbidity reflect more conservative best estimates.

One final tip for increasing the effectiveness of the CPT. Don't forget to consider nonmonetary contract benefits. For example, TLTC polices usually include a care coordination benefit. Families find that care coordination is very helpful in terms of next steps when a claim arises.

How about where to buy a policy. Policies are sold individually, to couples, or through employment.

Takeaway:

All options should be on the table. The more you personally explore an option—including past history and current offerings—the more you will find options that may be right for you. Then, dig in and get personalized details from a professional.

CHAPTER 26

The Evolving Worksite Extended and Long-Term Care Marketplace

Aside from working individually with an agent, you may be able to buy a policy as part of the supplemental benefits offered through your employer.

The worksite market has expanded to include hybrid/combo/linked sales as well as individual policies and group certificates sold with discounts and/or underwriting concessions to qualifying groups of people based on common employment. Fortunately, Jackson's friend Doug is able to share his experience with worksite LTC.

> *"My employer offered worksite long-term care coverage. I took advantage of the offer, bought a policy, and have the deductions taken right out of my paycheck. I elected to include a 3 percent inflation benefit on my policy to keep up with increasing medical and care expenses. I am no longer with that employer. I took a different position*

and moved back here, but the policy is still in force. I now pay the premiums directly. Actually, I have them automatically withdrawn from my bank account. I'm pretty happy to report that my maximum daily benefit amount has grown thanks to the inflation benefit."

"So you found the process pretty easy, Doug? Even after leaving that particular employer, they didn't drop you?" Jodi asks.

"Nope. I did some research before buying the policy. I didn't like what I read about employed caregivers and I didn't want anyone to be caught in that position. Doug holds up a sheet of paper. "I brought a clipping for to-night's session from a Transamerica Retirement Center survey of workers. 'Twenty-eight percent of workers are currently serving and/or have served as a caregiver for a relative or friend during the course of their working career. Current research about the impact of being an 'employed caregiver' foretells an alarming future reality that may very negatively impact not only us but genera-tions above and beneath us as well.

Among those who have served as a caregiver during their working careers, the vast majority have made one or more changes to their work as a result of becoming a caregiver, including using vacation, sick days, and/or personal days off (37 percent); missing days of work (36 percent); and reducing hours (20 percent)."[72]

"I personally did not qualify for a promotion due to caring for my parents," Jodi admits. "Along with short-and long-term financial repercussions, I certainly also experienced fallout at work and emotional stress at home.

Now that my parents have a funded plan in place, I am no longer continuously stressed and dreading personal or professional consequences."

Curious, Nicole asks," So, why don't more employers offer long-term care insurance as a supplemental employee benefit?"

That's a valid question. I suspect some of it has to do with how it is presented as an employee benefit. It's important to capture the priorities of the owners of small companies or human resources departments and/or the executive leadership of larger companies who generally decide on which employee benefits to offer. The priorities of owners or the leadership must be included and make sense to the decision maker, such as the positive effect of lowering the impact of absenteeism or presenteeism, which is being physically present but mentally absent.

Over many years of working in this area, I became associated with brokers/agents that developed tried-and-true methodologies. They have a proven track record that assures the employer that things will run smoothly. In some cases, they offer additional WellCare programs, which are accessible to all employees whether they buy coverage or not, as long as the employer puts a long-term care program in place.

There are a couple of considerations the employer may have before agreeing to offer employees a worksite LTC program. Is there a group design that fits the employer and their employees? Who works with employees before, during, and after the plan is put in place? Who works with newly eligible employees? Are spouses and/or extended family members eligible for coverage? Can premiums be payroll deducted? An important discussion may center around tax incentives.

There are three basic plan designs for employer-sponsored long-term care benefit programs: 100% voluntary programs where the employee pays the entire premium; core-group plans where the employer pays for a base plan and individuals can buy additional coverage; and executive carve-out plans where the employer can select participants, select a plan, and pay the premiums for an established group of selected employees. A good brokerage firm will manage the entire process from the introduction of the employer conversation, presentation of the plan options, education of employees, installment processes to minimize work for HR or in the case of smaller businesses, the person in charge of insurances, and the follow-up for new employees.

In terms of the individual pricing of a long-term care insurance policy in a worksite setting, the cost is determined in much the same way as when you purchase individual coverage. Your individual premium is based in part on your age, gender, the number of years that you expect to be paid a benefit, your health, the elimination period you select, the maximum daily and lifetime maximum dollar benefit, and whether you include an inflation rider or other riders. Basically, the cost will depend on the coverage you choose. Logically, the younger you elect coverage, the less expensive it will be if one assumes you would also be in better health. In some worksite cases, there is a discount and/or a measure of relaxed underwriting for which individuals in the group may qualify.

Unique Tax Advantages

DEDUCTIBILITY

LTC Insurance [LTCi] is considered Health Insurance.

Any premium paid on behalf of owners/employees, their spouses and dependents, retirees, and their spouses is **fully deductible** as a business expense.

Premiums may be paid from Health Savings Accounts (HSA).

INCOME REPORTING

Any premium paid on behalf of owners'/employees, their spouses and dependents, and retirees and their spouses is not considered imputed income to the insured.

TAXATION OF BENEFITS

Benefits recieved from Tax-Qualified (TQ) reimbursement contracts are **tax free.**

Benefits recieved from Tax-Qualified indemnity contracts in excess of $400/day (2021) are taxable to the extent the benefits recieved are not justified by actual expenses.

DISCRIMINATION RULES

With respect to employer contributory arrangements, the employer is not subject to anti-discrimination rules. Employer-paid TQ LTCi policies are NOT covered under the Employee Retirement Income Security Act of 1974 [ERISA].

An employer's ability to offer benefits on a disparate basis assumes the LTC insurance is not being offered through a plan that requires discrimination testing, e.g., Section 125 cafeteria plan or a pension plan. Currently, LTC insurance is not an eligble benefit under Section 125.

For subchapter C corporations. With respect to LTCi premium deductibility for owners of other corporate entities, different rules apply.
HSAs can only be established in conjunction with high-deductible health insurance plans and are not to be confused with Flexible Spending Accounts (FSAs).
For subchapter C corporations. With respect to income reporting for owners of other corporate entities, different rules apply.
A taxpayer seeking advice with regard to a particular situation must consult with his or her independent tax advisor.
Courtesy James Shea, CLTC, AVP, Marketing & Operations, Advanced Resources Marketing, JShea@armltc.com (800)269-2622

A very different program available to workers in the state of Washington (WA) is a first-in-the-nation publicly funded program that provides Washington state working residents an opportunity to vest into a basic level of LTC benefits. The program will be financed by WA workers who will pay a premium assessment (in the form of a tax on W-2 earnings) through payroll deductions. Employees who attest that they have long-term care insurance purchased prior to the established November 1, 2021 cut-off date were able to apply for an exemption from the premium tax. The program is designed to provide eligible residents with no maximum daily benefit, with a maximum lifetime limit of $36,500 (adjusted for inflation), to pay for long-term care services for eligible residents who qualify for benefits. Benefits will be available to qualifying individuals beginning on January 1, 2025. Individuals in Washington should consult their own legal or tax professional for specifics and information concerning this first publicly funded program.

Additional states are considering various ideas and solutions since, as we reviewed in this book, the need to prepare is very pressing.

The expression "adjusted for inflation" is often mentioned in discussing extended or long-term care. It is worth respecting one of the CPT's rules of seeking definitions and meaning of words as used in the context of specific insurance products. An inflation increase or an inflation rider is generally designed to protect the value of the dollar benefit from being eroded over time. It is a feature in which the value of the dollar benefits increase by a predefined percentage at specific time periods to help policyholders make sure that the benefits they receive can keep up with general price levels.

Takeaway:

Worksite programs play a key role in helping employees access long-term care benefits that fit their needs and lifestyles. Purchasing or paying for future benefits at the worksite should involve education and advice. Don't hesitate to ask questions!

CHAPTER 27

Whole Life and Universal Life Insurance

While TLTC and worksite LTC products may be specifically designed to provide coverage for long-term care, other insurances may provide funding. Whole life insurance may provide permanent death benefit coverage for the life of the insured. The cash accounts are guaranteed to grow based on insurance company calculations; while with universal life policies, cash grows, depending on the policy, based on current interest rates.[73] Cash-value life insurance usually has a level premium in which money dedicated to cash accumulation decreases over time, and money paid for insurance increases, due to the higher cost to insure you as you age.

Premiums are split up into three pools: one portion for the death benefit, one portion for the insurer's costs and profits, and one for the cash value.

The CPT gets together and Jackson wants to explain that he has a whole life insurance policy, but unlike Grandpa he sees it as an asset as much as a legacy.

"When Mom and I first got married," Jackson says, looking affectionately at Jodi, "I wanted to be sure that if something happened to me, she would have money to support herself . . . and later you kids. So, I bought a whole life insurance policy. The cash-value portion of my policy accrues tax-deferred interest, and I can withdraw a limited amount of cash from my policy. In the policy I have, I can take a nontaxable cash-value withdrawal up to my policy basis, which is the amount of premiums I've paid into the policy. Mom and I discussed the possibility of using this as an option to pay for unexpected care costs."

Policy loans are borrowed against the death benefit, and the insurance company uses the policy as collateral for the loan. Life insurance companies add interest to the balance, which accrues whether the loan is paid monthly or not. Jackson will need to go over details with his agent and understand all the pros and cons of this option.

Takeaway:

Don't overlook assets such as whole life policies and universal life polices, which may be a good fit. Aside from accumulated cash value, a new version of variable universal life insurance includes riders designed to provide a living benefit for extended or long-term care needs.

CHAPTER 28

What's Happening in the Hybrid/Combo/ Linked-Benefit Marketplace

As we move to a discussion about hybrid/combo/linked marketplace products, insurance lingo tends to become even more specialized, if not convoluted. What name an insurer assigns to their product or how they market it under that name or category can be confusing. Similar to other emerging product lines, I guess we will have to allow the industry some time to standardize terminology to keep up with the innovation of products and services.

That being said, it's helpful to break up these options into smaller digestible pieces. It involves a good deal of information. And that is good news. As we said, one size does not fit all!

Currently, each insurer may use one of four names for similar but different products: combination, linked, asset based, or hybrid. No matter what the product is called, what is important is what the product does or does not do in terms of your personal situation and objectives.

The CPT seems to be willing to tackle the complexity—but start off on a light note! Their banter reminds us that members of the CPT play different roles, have different relationships with one another, and have different skill sets.

After announcing that the devil is in the details and that this section includes several options, Erik reminds his mother, "Nicole is the detail person and I prefer the big picture view." Grinning, Erik adds, "It works really well for us when we deal with options for parental issues. So, if I don't ask specific questions, it doesn't mean I am lost or not paying attention."

"OK, Erik," Jodi says, her tone serious while her face reveals her amusement. "Dad and I respect your division of labor! Speaking of a division, here is how I suggest we divide up this more complex topic. We will schedule a series of four calls. This call will focus on the foundation and expansion of the hybrid/combo/linked-benefit marketplace. Our second call will review life insurance with long-term care riders, and our third call will focus on annuities to which riders can attach. The fourth call will focus on various riders currently available to pair up with various products."

"Sounds good." Erik says, then he asks, "So, why did carriers create these types of policies since there are TLTC policies still available?"

Good question! Even though newer TLTC policies are less susceptible to premium increases, they still don't address one of the most frequent objections to purchasing TLTC, which is if you don't need long-term care, you lose all the money you paid in premiums. Although TLTC carriers offer return-of-premium options, they can be rather expensive.

Hearing consumer objections and reactions to premium increases on the TLTC products, insurers began to introduce products that offer more guarantees. Then, the sudden nightmare and uncertainly about long-term effects on people's health brought on by the COVID-19 and associated variants, the persistence of low interest rates, and continually increasing health-care costs drove insurers back to the drawing board. Understandably, for the sake of sustainability, newer and updated products take into account changing economic and health environments.

In response to the reality of the marketplace, some insurers are creating products that incorporate flexibility in their plan design and investment opportunities for younger purchasers. The first of the millennial cohort turned 40 years old in 2021, and they have growing insurance and risk coverage needs. At that age, they have a long investment horizon and may want to take advantage of stock market growth potential. Insurers are responding with products that speak to lifestyle and investment opportunities aimed at a younger market. Awareness is still an issue for the industry, especially for the younger generations.

Luckily, Erik and Nicole learned the advantages of planning from their involvement with the CPT.

Erik comments, "We came close to experiencing lots of difficult, nonreversible consequences for all of us. Nicole and I are two generations down from our grandparents, but we still felt the emotional impact. I suspect the financial impact of so many people being unprepared will be

*felt via state and federal budgets, which will impact all
of us financially."*

*"Too true," Jackson remarks. "Which is one of the reasons
carriers are creating these types of policies that combine
two types of insurance products. It's in response to consumer demand and a desire to broaden the marketplace.
The hope is that more people will be interested in planning and these newer iterations of policies will provide
more people affordable coverage that works with their
objectives."*

*Nicole says, "Well, you would think that seeing and hear-
ing in the news what is coming with illnesses, an aging
population, and the overwhelming difficulty of finding
qualified staffing for hospitals and other facilities, health-
care aides, first responders, and emergency services that
everyone would certainly be open to at least a discussion
about how to plan for themselves and those they love."*

*When I bought my policy at work, I felt I did a little
nursing home avoidance planning," Doug reveals. "It's
good that insurers are creating products that can serve a
wider swath of Americans."*

You might be wondering why insurers didn't create these types of
products sooner. Let's just say it took an act to encourage them to act.
The Pension Protection Act (PPA) of 2006 provided new tax benefits
that encouraged carriers to create these new types of products.

In terms of insurance or marketing lingo, a combination, or
combo, product is generally considered the most generic of all the
various types. It's an umbrella term and may include LTC riders on
life insurance, linked-benefit LTC, and annuity-based LTC coverage
as well as chronic illness riders on life insurance.

Linked-benefit LTC describes products that link or employ two pools of money. In some cases, life insurance is linked to an LTC rider that may also be linked to an extension of benefits (EOB) rider, which provides the second pool of LTC benefits. This pool is *only* available to the policy owner for qualified LTC needs. When the LTC rider benefits from the first benefit pool are exhausted, only then does the EOB rider start paying.

Others carriers developed LTC hybrid products, which refer to policies that look and feel like traditional LTC policies but whose chassis, or base, is a financial product—thus why they are considered hybrid.

As mentioned before, one important rule is to look at the words as defined in the policy to understand what the policy actually provides or describes. Let's look at the term *rider*. A rider is essentially an additional benefit added to an insurance policy that may or may not require an additional premium payment. Riders can customize an insurance policy to address specific needs or concerns.

Some policies allow the addition of more than one rider to a single policy. For example, adding an inflation rider to an EOB rider in a hybrid LTC plus life insurance policy results in the maximum long-term care benefit being much greater than the death benefit of the life insurance policy.

Some things become clear when you examine which section of the Internal Revenue Code (IRC) governs the type of rider an insurer uses with the benefit; for example, they may use Section 7702B or IRC Section 101g. Since tax implications should be handled by your tax advisor, those details are beyond the scope of our overview.

There are significant differences in products, which is why I advise you to take a deep dive with a specialist once you have an overview of options that interest you. They will help you determine the direction that fits your needs. Remember, the name is not the determinate factor, the contract is.

Checking back in with the CPT, we see they are quickly absorbing the basics.

Doug has a playful sparkle in his eyes as he says, "Are these sometimes called twofers? Jackson and I were watching the game the other night, and we mentioned that we were looking into some policies for extended care coverage. One of our buddies said, "Oh, so are you considering a twofer? At first we thought he had switched topics and was talking about betting on the game!"

Everyone enjoys Doug's quip. "I have heard that expression as well. My understanding is that twofers refer to a contract that covers more than one risk; in this case, it refers to a policy that offsets some extended or long-term care risks as well as premature death risks. If care is not needed, these policies will pay a death benefit, or in the case of an annuity, a stream of income payments."

"Thanks for that info, Doug." Jodi wraps up the session. "Well that's our introduction to this growing marketplace. Next week, we will dive into some details on hybrid and linked life insurance policies. Since Doug has created his own moniker for these products that cover two risks, we will let him start things off at our next meeting."

Takeaway:

Whether you are older or younger, one of the advantages of participating in the CPT is it allows you to be an active listener and get acquainted with the scope of available, evolving, and new options.

CHAPTER 29

What Are Twofers and Double Twofers, and How Can They Help?

After greetings are exchanged, Doug starts off the CPT conversation by reminding everyone that he was assigned the twofer topic. Trying to suppress a smile, he feigns discontentment. "That's what I get for making a joke about such a serious topic."

Jodi throws him a phony reprimanding expression and playfully adds, "The stage is yours, Doug."

"Thanks, Jodi! Twofers, as I refer to them, are products that are designed to serve two needs or offset two risks. Depending on what product the insurance carrier develops, these products may offer tax-free reimbursements for qualified long-term care expenses; tax-free death benefits to heirs if some portion of the benefit is not used for

long-term care expenses; and, in some cases, a potential return of your premium if you change your mind."

Having described what twofers do, Doug continues with product design. "All riders, which are add-on features, are attached to a base plan and are decided at the time of purchase—unless there is no charge for the rider. That doesn't make it free. The charge is factored into the total premium costs."

There are three common forms of double twofers where the addition of a rider to a life insurance policy provides extended or LTC coverage:

- Life insurance with an LTC accelerated death benefit (ADB) rider
- LTC plus life insurance with an extension of benefits (EOB) rider
- Life insurance with a chronic illness (CI) rider

Depending on your budget and risk tolerance, traditional or hybrid policies can be reviewed in terms of your desired level of certainty concerning premium stability and/or guaranteed benefits.

Importance of Guarantees to Premium Risk Level Tolerance

Certainty of	Traditional LTC	Guaranteed LTC + Life Linked Plans	LTC + Life Indexed Universal Life Plans	LTC + Life Variable Universal Life LTC Plans
Premiums	No	Yes	Yes	Probably No
Benefits	Yes	Yes	No	No

Tom Riekse, "How Low Interest Rates Are Changing LTC Insurance Products, April 22.2021 https://lecp.naifa.org/how-low-interest-rates-are-changing-ltc-insurance-products

Not every insurer who offers life insurance offers a long-term care rider or guaranteed benefit premiums. Generally, life insurance carriers who offer an accelerated death benefit (ADB) rider have policies that often pay only one benefit, either a long-term care benefit or a death benefit, or a lesser combination of the two, but never both in their entirety.

Erik, who is a car enthusiast, comments, "It sounds sort of like car manufacturers who create different models on a chassis. They build the base and then add or subtract different features."

Doug shares Erik's enthusiasm. "Yes, Erik, I can see that as an overarching concept!" He decides to leave the discussion about add-ons for another day. "Staying on topic, it's important to remember that the first and foremost reason that people usually buy life insurance is that at least one person, possibly more, depends on them financially. It may also be used in estate planning designs."

Jackson relates this point to his own situation. "That means if you absolutely need the life insurance to be in place as part of family protection, a legacy, or as part of spousal protection in retirement planning, that consideration may mean that, initially, someone may not select life insurance as the base product where the death benefit is diminished by the living benefit. Since Jodi and I already have life insurance in place, that isn't a major concern for us if we select a hybrid policy."

"So here comes the part where I explain why Jodi commandeered me for this product option. We know the death benefit is designed to take care of loved ones if someone dies, but—and this important—this living

benefit is designed to avoid negative consequences for the family, or a friend, if the insured doesn't die."

Nicole replies, "So, Doug, these twofer policies cover two risks, one being premature death and the other being extended care needs of the policyholder. Those certainly help family and friends. But, Doug, they are really double twofers.

"First, the policy helps avoid certain unwanted consequences for the insured's family via the death benefit."

"Second, the policy can provide care funding so family members or friends don't forcibly become caregivers."

Nicole pauses, then continues. "And three, these policies also provide funding for the personal care wishes of the insured person, so they can choose how, where, and who takes care of them."

"Fourth, the policy also diminishes stress and offers dignity to the policyholder so they don't have to feel like a burden to the family."

"So, they are actually double twofers!"

Everyone appreciates the dramatic delivery, rather unusual for Nicole. Doug happily concedes, "Double twofers. I love it, Nicole!"

It is good to see the CPT enjoying themselves as they internalize and personalize the information. Speaking of information, the two types of riders mentioned previously—the accelerated death benefit rider and the extension of benefits rider—require some explanation.

Let's take a closer look at life insurance with a long-term care acceleration death benefit (ADB) rider. If the rider is "free" of charge, no additional money is added to the cost of the policy for the rider. If there is a qualifying long-term care claim, it simply reduces the death benefit that the beneficiary would be entitled to receive. If long-term care services are not needed or if all of the death benefit is not used up to pay for long-term care expenses, the remaining death benefit is paid out to the beneficiaries upon the death of the insured.

Here's a simple example: A $120,000 life insurance policy with a four-year ADB rider might provide for a maximum benefit of $2,500, to be paid each month for forty-eight months while the insured is using qualified long-term care services. The amount being accelerated will reduce the death benefit on the contract dollar for dollar. The insurer may require that a small death benefit remain, so that may change the payable benefit. A logical question you might ask is, "If I exhaust the entire available death benefit by accessing the ADB rider, what happens if I still need care?"

For some individuals, it's a valid concern. As a result, some insurers responded by offering an extension of benefits (EOB) rider .

Linked-benefit life insurance with an EOB rider features two distinct benefit pools. Adding an EOB rider means that LTC benefits may be paid out even after the death benefit has been depleted. As we saw previously, the first benefit pool available for qualified extended or long-term care needs is created by the acceleration of the death benefit rider. In the example, there is a four-year benefit payout of $120,000. Let's assume the insured exhausts that benefit. Let's further assume that the insured continues to be on claim and continues to qualify for care. In that case, benefits will be paid from the second pool, which is the EOB rider pool. Depending on the insurer, the second pool may be two or three times more than the policy's death benefit. Now, let's add an inflation benefit to the second pool. Now, the benefit pool may grow to be $360,000 or more. It is very important to understand that the second pool, the EOB rider pool, may *only* be used for extended or long-term care benefits. It does *not* pay out as a death benefit.

If care is needed, the triggers to pay for benefits are generally the same as for TLTC. The individual must need substantial help with two or more activities of daily living (ADL) or have severe cognitive impairment that requires continual supervision to prevent them from harming themselves or others. The activities of daily living are bathing, dressing, toileting, continence, transferring, and eating. Although we generally associate these care needs with aging, individuals may need help with these activities after an accident, stroke, major surgery, complications of a chronic illness, or other serious conditions.

Since not everyone may want or qualify for life insurance, some insurers offer a second option to serve as a financial base for extended or long-term care riders. While life insurance provides a tax-free benefit upon death of the insured, an annuity is designed to provide a steady income stream similar to a pension plan. To protect that steady income source from depletion by extended or long-term care needs, a rider can be added.

Takeaway:

The reality of double twofers or any policies that serve to help both the care recipient and caregiver cannot be fully appreciated until you have the experience. Hopefully, you plan and experience the positive effects of preparation and ownership.

CHAPTER 30

Annuities as an Asset Base for Extended or LTC Riders

In a sense, an annuity is like reverse life insurance. Instead of insuring against death, annuities are designed to protect against "longevity risk," the risk that you will outlive your income and savings.

Basically, an annuity is a contract between you and an insurance company or similar financial institution under which, in exchange for a lump sum or ongoing premium payments, the insurance company agrees to make regular payments for either the rest of your life or for a predetermined number of years.

This important option for covering extended or long-term care has some real advantages, the least of which is a potential tax benefit. Previously, if the insured took an annuity withdrawal to cover costs associated with long-term care needs, they dealt with the associated ordinary income, gains-first tax treatment and paid taxes accordingly.[74]

On the other hand, there are the annuity expenses and fees, including mortality and expense (M&E) fees and administrative fees.

These charges pay for any insurance guarantees that are automatically included in the annuity as well as the selling and administrative expenses of the contract.

Annuities can be classified as either immediate, deferred, fixed, variable, or indexed.

One of the biggest attractions of annuities is that the growth earned on the single sum or ongoing payments isn't taxable right away. This feature, called deferred growth, means you don't owe any taxes on an annuity's earnings until you actually receive the money. The period in which you start receiving money back from the insurance company is known as the annuitization phase.

To summarize, the annuitization phase is simply the time period when the insurance company is paying you, as opposed to the accumulation phase when you are paying the insurance company. Each distribution is composed of both growth and a return of premium, which is a repayment of your initial investment. Since you already paid taxes on the money that you used to pay premiums, the initial investment isn't taxable, but you will pay taxes on the growth.[75]

Similar to what is happening in the life insurance marketplace, annuity carriers stay abreast of current financial and medical events. Due to long-term uncertainties created by the COVID-19 pandemic, coupled with the prolonged low interest rate environment, insurers may modify, withdraw, or restore certain guarantees in response to the realities of the marketplace.

If you purchase an annuity as part of a retirement plan using pretax money, it is called a qualified annuity. Because no income taxes have been paid on the premium, all payments from a qualified annuity are taxable income when received.

For those of us who are visual learners, this chart helps explain qualified versus nonqualified annuities.[76]

Qualified vs. Non-Qualified Funding

Type	Purchased With	Annual Cap on Purchase	Withdrawal Funds Taxed	Distribution Requirement
Qualified	Pre-tax funds (tax-favored retirement money, such as IRA contributions)	Yes, the IRS limits how much of your income you may invest annually	Yes, payouts are taxed as income	You must begin withdrawing funds by age 70 1/2
Non-Qualified	After-tax funds (money on which taxes have been paid)	No cap	Only your earnings are taxed as income; principal is not.	No requirement

Elaine Silvestrini, financially revied by Rubina Houssain, CFP®, "Qualified vs. Non-Qualified Annuities,
https://www.annuity.org/annuities/taxation/qualified-vs-nonqualified/

Depending on personal selection, either annuity funding design could provide income to pay for some of the expenses associated with long-term care. Similar to life insurance, the concern is, what would be left for lifestyle or family needs once you use that income for LTC expenses? Adding an extended or long-term care rider to an annuity ameliorates that concern.

Some insurers, agents, or advisors may refer to an annuity to which a rider is added as the asset base. Originally, riders were attached to single-pay premium annuities. Referring to a single-pay annuity as an asset, the expression *asset base with rider* became popular. Over time, insurers offered policies with multiple pay periods, so the term became less prevalent.

Usually, an annuity pays one monthly benefit amount. But if you ever need long-term care, some annuities adjust the income payout in the form of a higher monthly benefit that's a multiple of the premiums you've paid. Let's say you are scheduled to receive a monthly income payment of $2,500; if you qualify and are approved for long-term care benefits under the long-term care rider, the payment may double to $5,000 per month. The increased payments are typically available for a set number of years.

After reviewing the basic types of annuities, the CPT starts to compile a list of questions to discuss with their agent or advisor.

Doug is curious if this option is a serious contender for his friend's coverage. "If you both qualify and need LTC benefits, does the LTC rider cover both of you?

Erik's love of cars comes in handy. "Car insurers offer different discounts when you have multiple vehicles or drivers. Is it similar if couples buy a single policy together? Is there a couple's discount?"

Doug asks, "How does the death benefit pay heirs if the policyholder dies and the long-term care benefits haven't been used?"

"My question" Jodi says, "is if I am using the increased LTC benefit for a couple of years and then stop, does the benefit carry over to a second incident if I again qualify?"

Erik recalls they didn't define an elimination period. "And what about an elimination period? How do they define it if there is one? Does it need to be satisfied twice if you stop receiving a benefit and then qualify a second time?"

This is a really good use of the CPT members' time. They are coming up with questions to ask, broadening their overall financial education, and working as a team. Moreover, Jodi and Jackson will benefit from the CPT's insights and questions.

While Erik and Nicole are focused on their parent's planning, do they, the younger members of the CPT, gain anything from spending time and energy on a topic that must seem very remote in terms of their time line?

Erik and Nicole have odd expressions on their faces. Jodi hesitates but decides to ask if there is an issue. She thought creating a list of questions was a positive thing to do. Their expressions say otherwise.

Nicole says, "We agree that reviewing the options will help us feel more confident and ask more personalized questions when working with a professional. So, let me thank you for that, for both of us, right now." Jodi is visibly moved, if not confused, by the unexpected appreciation.

Erik elaborates on the surprising direction of the conversation. "Honestly, Mom, we were not that interested in being part of another CPT after we got Grandma and Grandpa's plan done."

Nicole adds, "Erik and I were trying to figure out how to tell you and Dad, but the more we talked, the more we realized that our grandparents actually had a plan that they worked toward for years. They consistently paid their Medicare Advantage policy premium, invested their savings, served in the military, and built up the equity in their home. So the solution open to them, while it seemed new to the rest of us, had actually involved years of planning so they could age in the home they love. Finding the funding mechanism just took some investigation, and we determined which government programs would help and let go of an old concept about reverse mortgages.

"When you said that you and Dad wanted to redo the three simple steps to avoid being rushed into a solution that you may not like or want, we felt obligated," Nicole admits with a look of apology. "But we also wanted to be supportive," she added quickly.

"At the end of the day," Erik adds, "going through the steps have rewarded each of us."

Nicole continues, "We have enjoyed being included, value what we have learned, and now realize what to consider for ourselves. We simply had no idea extended or LTC was truly part of planning for a more secure financial future. Hopefully using a plan for care is way off in the future, but it may not be. We both need life insurance, and now we know we can consider a double twofer. Of equal importance, the process of discovering various options has helped us relax, take control, and decide what direction we want to go and what questions to ask to get us there."

Jackson, looking at his wife, realizes she is a bit overcome. He responds for both of them. "Thank you! Mom and I must admit that our motivation was to avoid creating havoc in your lives and, I suppose, in ours as well. Watching the impact on Mom that caring for her parents was having while she was trying to maintain her job, her finances, her sanity, and her health was something we didn't want for you." With a playful tone, Jackson adds, "Being caught in the sandwich generation is not a gift we want to give you kids."

Jackson's quip brings things back to a lighter tone. Faces brighten and everyone is ready to get back at it!

The CPT gets back to adding questions to the list. "Do you two still remember the questions you texted me?" Jodi asks.

"Yup! Are annuities underwritten like life insurance?" Nicole is still looking for details!

The CPT is asking really good questions. Generally, the underwriting on LTC annuities is less rigorous than for hybrid life/LTC and stand-alone TLTC policies. There may still be some medical underwriting in the form of five or six health questions. In any case, the insurance carrier still reserves the right to get medical records.

Erik asks the broader question, "Who is a good candidate for an annuity versus a TLTC policy?"

An annuity applicant with arthritis who has had two knee replacements may be a good candidate for this type of annuity since they may find it difficult to qualify for a TLTC policy.

Adding a continuation of benefits (COB) rider is good for people who are looking for lifetime or unlimited long-term care benefits, which are extremely expensive, if available, on TLTC policies.

You might wonder why someone would want a lifetime benefit.

The CPT is wondering the same thing. Stories about long-term care needs are becoming more and more prevalent! Nicole offers the group some insight.

"The dad of one of my college friends was diagnosed with early onset Alzheimer's disease. She described to me the sadness and the nightmare of when her dad first admitted that he wasn't quite "right." For a long time, her dad, along with everyone else, just tried to ignore it. As Mom has pointed out several times, aging or needing care is a tough subject to discuss. Everyone tried to pretend it would just get better or go away. It doesn't just go away, and they are looking at years of increasing costly care."

"How old was her dad?" Jackson asks, "What did they do?"

"He was young, in his early sixties. I think they went bankrupt, if not financially, then for sure emotionally.

The toll on my friend was huge." Dismay is evident on everyone's faces. "After a semester, she took a leave to help her mom with her dad. Eventually, they had to find a facility for him. It cut her to the core, not just because she was seeing her dad's mental health deteriorate, but she sort of lost her mom as well. The impact on her future is uncertain since I don't know if she returned to school or could afford to. I haven't thought about it for years. I'm not sure what the final outcome for her or her family was. She told me the disease is hereditary. Hopefully, she put a plan in place for herself, just in case. I think that unlimited coverage is probably something she would consider."

Erik says, "Wow, you hear about these types of situations, but I agree with my sister, the tendency is to push those thoughts away and just hope it doesn't happen in your family."

Jodi sighs. "Between accidents, long-lasting illnesses, debilitating diseases, Alzheimer's disease, and other forms of dementia increasing with the aging of the baby boomer population, it is safe to say that services and especially professional and supportive personnel for care needs are going to be pushed beyond the limit. While technology is racing to help with monitoring care, support nurses, doctors, and facility staff, help will probably be in short supply and expensive. And then, like Grandpa, some people find technology aids invasive, which can limit their effectiveness."

While certainly not limited to only older adults, it's often difficult to get a parent, sister, brother, close friend, and so on to discuss their health and possible care needs.

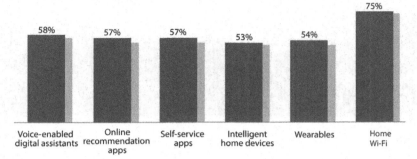

Consumers Likely to Buy or Increase Their Use of Technology

Voice-enabled digital assistants	Online recommendation apps	Self-service apps	Intelligent home devices	Wearables	Home Wi-Fi
58%	57%	57%	53%	54%	75%

https://insuranceblog.accenture.com/wp-content/uploads/2020/06/GASC_COVID-19-Six-post-pandemic-priorities-facing-insurers_CVID-19_BLOG3_Picture1.png accessed 6/16/20

Takeaway:

The insurance industry has truly created products to respond to the realities of accidents, illnesses, and aging. Don't be a victim of your circumstances. Instead reap the benefits of your planning decisions.

"The most common way people give up their power is by thinking they don't have any." (Alice Walker)

Technology

Telehealth and technology startups seem to be popping up each day, and established companies are also showing serious interest in such devices. Technology is making some real headway in the extended and LTC arena. Generations are becoming more connected through media technologies, wearables, actuarial science, and data science. Advanced devices apply artificial intelligence (AI), machine learning, and behavioral science–backed "nudges and alerts" to help users act on resulting insights and maintain personalized wellness habits. Home care and the potential for aging in place is continually improving through the use of robotics and interactive telehealth technologies to mediate the interaction between patients and medical professionals in real time.

Big data and computing power are exploding at exponential rates. The data collected will be vital to the predictive future of LTC insurance, positioning insurance companies as a valuable partner in helping consumers with both their wellness and insurance needs.

CHAPTER 31

Single Premium Immediate Annuity

Responding to the reality that consumers have many different needs, some carriers designed an annuity for income purposes only. A medically underwritten single premium immediate annuity (SPIA) helps fund immediate care needs with monthly payments guaranteed for life. While this income stream may be guaranteed for life, like all extended or long-term care options, it may not cover all costs associated with long-term care. As the name indicates, it differs from a deferred annuity, which begins payments at a future date chosen by the annuity owner.

A SPIA may also be called an income annuity, or simply an immediate annuity. When you purchase a SPIA, you trade a large, lump-sum premium payment up front for extended, periodic payouts from an insurance company or a similar institution. The lump sum may come from money that has already been taxed or from pre-taxed money, such as from a 401(k) or IRA. It's best to seek tax advice right from the start to determine the effect of taxed or nontaxed payouts. With the guidance of your tax advisor, you select the type of interest rate (fixed or variable) along with the duration and frequency of annuitization payouts. An immediate annuity pays the owner or annuitant a guaranteed income starting almost immediately. You may also have the option of continuing payouts to beneficiaries if death occurs before a certain period of time has elapsed. In terms of extended care or long-term care, SPIAs are used when guaranteed payments are needed to provide services for care.

This type of policy is attractive for someone with a health-related condition, such as heart disease, alcoholism, leukemia, or cirrhosis of the liver, that might shorten their life.

The underwriting is unique. Instead of proving you are in good health, the applicant is actually required to provide documentation to support their heath condition diagnosis. As you might suspect, the insurer may further investigate the applicant's health history and may include a request that the applicant undergo a medical exam. The SPIA underwriting allows insurers to take into account an applicant's lifestyle, such as, smoking, drinking, or drugs, as well as other risk factors, such as a bad driving record, engagement in dangerous hobbies, and medical history to determine life expectancy and therefore the rate for scheduled payouts.

This annuity has some unique advantages:

- The more ill the applicant, the higher the payments.
- Immediate annuities don't have any account management or account maintenance charges.
- Once established, an immediate annuity requires no maintenance or work.
- It is easy to calculate how much money will be available to pay for monthly care costs.
- The reliability of a SPIA may be preferable to stock market value fluctuations.

Depending on the immediacy of the extended or long-term care situation, an impaired risk rider can be added to an annuity. If you have a health condition or injury that is expected to shorten your life span, the insurer will use a rated age instead of their chronological age for the impaired risk rider. The rider is the provision that will accelerate the income payments in the annuity, most commonly a SPIA. Simply stated, depending on the health condition, you will receive higher income payments or a lower premium based on your expected life expectancy. While most annuities are not medically underwritten, if you decide to add the impaired risk rider, your annuity will be medically underwritten.

At the time of purchase, how long you will live is an unknown. There is a possibility that you will live longer than the insurance company expects, and will, therefore, collect more in income payments than you paid in premiums.

Members of the CPT are discovering products responsive to different consumer needs. It comes as no surprise that additional riders and add-on benefits tailored to specific care needs have been and continue to be introduced. According to the CPT agenda, some of the additional riders are the topic of the next Zoom call.

Takeaway:

Many insurers target different health-care needs brought on by different lifestyles, family health history, and financial circumstances. Peace of mind comes with discovering, preparing, and planning for your specific need.

CHAPTER 32

How Riders and Add-On Benefits Can Help with Specific Care Needs

As the industry engages in developing products in response to marketplace demand, they must meet established regulatory, legislative, and tax code requirements. Employing different sections of the IRS code, insurers have developed riders that can be added to insurance products, which are responsive to specific care needs. Let's join in on the CPT Zoom call in progress.

Critical Illness and Terminal Illness Riders

Jackson announces that riders are his assignment. "Aside from long-term care riders, there are terminal illness riders, critical illness riders, and chronic illness riders. It's important not to confuse one rider with another.

Critical illness riders differ from chronic illness riders. Critical illness insurance was developed in 1996, as people realized that surviving a heart attack or stroke could leave them with insurmountable medical bills. Critical illness insurance provides additional coverage for medical emergencies like heart attack, stroke, or cancer. It's fair to say that critical illness riders are more responsive to immediate needs as opposed to chronic or long-term care needs."

"For me, it's pretty easy to distinguish between terminal illness and critical illness," Erik says. "My understanding is that while both terms refer to serious medical conditions, the basic difference is that a critical illness refers to a specified serious injury, illness, or medical episode." Erik's somber tone indicates he has firsthand knowledge. "My friend Pete's mom became critically ill. She had a stroke that resulted in a permanent neurological deficit, meaning that even after good medical treatment, she can't manage on her own. Pete and his dad had to organize ongoing care. He said they were relieved that at least it wasn't a terminal illness diagnosis, which would have meant that his mom's illness would lead to death, likely within six to twenty-four months."

"I remember being very shocked by his mom's sudden illness," Jodi adds. "It came out of nowhere. She always seemed like such a healthy person. We used to go to the same gym. Hopefully, they have extended or long-term care insurance to help with the ongoing medical and care bills."

Looking at everyone's concerned expressions, Jackson mutters, "Well, you just never know. I am grateful that we don't have that kind of sad reality kicking us into gear. While there is no easy way to emotionally handle that sort of thing, it does speak to how much easier arranging ongoing care is if you prepare in advance for an unexpected event!"

Chronic Illness Rider

It would be wonderful to think of Erik's friend's situation as a one-off. But, that's not the case. As people face health issues, connected to aging or not, protection becomes more relevant. Life insurance with a chronic illness (CI) rider may be a good fit. A chronic illness can generally be defined as a condition with no medical cure, such as heart disease, certain cancers, Parkinson's disease, or multiple sclerosis. Chronic illnesses create an ongoing need that may last for years. Traditionally, policies offering CI riders only paid accelerated death benefit payments for a qualifying permanent condition. Recently, some of the newer contracts have removed the requirement. Have your agent check out this detail in the contract.

You should also ask the advisor or agent under which Internal Revenue Code (IRC) the rider is filed since there can be differences in the tax treatment. Aside from that important distinction, other differences surface when examining actual contract language. LTC rider regulations require that consumer protection provisions be included. CI riders are not required to include them, although some do.

For example, let's say Nicole's friend's dad who suffers from Alzheimer's disease has a policy. His policy includes an unintentional lapse provision and a reinstatement provision. Those two provisions are designed to address the concern that at the very time when he needs to activate the CI rider or LTC rider, he forgets to pay the policy premium because of his Alzheimer's disease. The policy reinstatement provision allows him or someone he designated to reinstate the policy without having to undergo underwriting again, which obviously could be a huge hurdle.

"Jackson and I have a friend, Brian, who is a successful retirement advisor." Jackson nods his agreement and Jodi continues. "Naturally, he made sure his parents had long-term care coverage in place. His dad started to suffer from dementia but hid it from the family. My understanding is that it's pretty typical. Brian, his dad, and his family were in denial. Anyway, his dad didn't pay the insurance premium, or as I understand it, he continued paying some bills but stopped paying others. The insurance policy went unpaid. The coverage lapsed. Thankfully, the policy contained a third-party notification clause, so after a couple of months, the insurer reached out to Brian. Fortunately, he contacted the carrier within the specified time period to provide proof that the condition caused the policy lapse."

Nicole looking pensive says, "I see why it is important to have an agent or advisor differentiate between the two riders in terms of consumer protections, among other things. But I am still a bit confused as to why there needs to be both long-term care and chronic illness riders? Chronic illnesses create an ongoing need that may last for years and long-term care needs can last for years. Is this another case of semantics?"

No, it's not semantics! It's more like different strokes for different folks. Chronic illnesses are on the rise in the United States. If you are tailoring the product selection to the person and not the other way around, either one of those two riders may be the right fit for people in different health situations.

CHRONIC DISEASES IN AMERICA

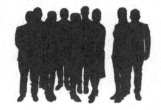

6 IN 10

Adults in the US
have a **chronic
disease**

4 IN 10

Adults in the US
have a **two
or more**

Jackson offers an example for the CPT members, who are still struggling with why both types of riders are available.

"This is how I understand it. While a broken hip with healing complications may qualify for benefits under an LTC rider, it probably would not qualify under a chronic illness rider. However, if the broken hip complications put you in a wheelchair for the rest of your life, your condition is now chronic and the rider may pay you benefits."

The CPT members are fast becoming knowledgeable consumers!

There are important details to discuss with your agent, advisor, or tax consultant concerning the design used to add chronic illness riders to a policy. There are three common designs for chronic illness riders: dollar for dollar, lien, and discounted. The cost of the riders can be funded through separate rider premiums or by applying cost of insurance (COI) charges against the policy value.

The introduction of these riders expanded available planning options.[77] As insurers continue to innovate in response to an evolving market, they continue to introduce new riders or modify existing ones.

For example, a newly introduced benefit attached to a universal life insurance linked benefit product is the transitional care assistance (TCA) benefit that helps clients transition from informal to formal care. Another is the long-term care benefit rider (LTCBR), which combines two riders. Rather than separate the accelerated death benefit (ADB) and extension of benefits (EOB) riders, the LTCBR allows for a streamlined contract structure and consistent pricing between the benefit period options. In response to consumer demand, insurers are adding aging-in-place riders. One insurer has added an amendment that provides clients additional benefit flexibility with access to receipt-free cash to help cover informal care needs at home, allowing for spouses to provide care. By offering less expensive limited-care options, the industry is reaching out to more and more consumers.

Takeaway:

The Care Guide should be an indicator of which type of care needs may arise in the future. Pairing the Care Guide with personal research and reading, and discussing options with your CPT, will lead to the best fit for your social and financial situation. Uncover your choices!

CHAPTER 33

Limited-Term Care Options

Short-Term Care Policies

Product innovation, along with awareness of services and costs, leads the CPT to the next option. Costs are always a major consideration in proper planning. A short-term care (STC) policy is a great option for someone who has health issues and is not insurable for TLTC but still wants coverage. One of our CPT members is caught in this scenario and looking for help.

> *Doug asks Jackson if he can meet him to grab a coffee. They settle into a corner of the café. Doug thanks Jackson for meeting him, explaining that he doesn't want to discuss this at home since it is about his father-in-law. He doesn't want to upset his wife.*

"I envy you, Jackson. You got your in-laws settled into a plan to deal with aging and the pressures of extended and long-term care needs."

"Thanks, Doug. What's on your mind? You look worried."

"Do you know if there is anything for someone who can't afford, qualify, or will not consider any of the insurance options we already discussed?"

"He won't consider any options that we discussed with Jodi's parents? We can review government programs, community services, or using the home as an asset to access income."

Doug shakes his head, "They rent their place, and he doesn't have much in savings, so a SPIA is probably out. He also says he won't consider government aid."

"I see."

"Worse than that, my wife refuses to push him, but her dad is going to need care. He has some serious issues. I suspect this won't be a case of long-term care, but even in the short term he isn't prepared for the cost of care services."

This is not an uncommon scenario. This is where a short-term care policy may be a viable option.

An STC policy is generally available for individuals between ages fifty and eighty-nine to cover gaps in Medicare coverage or as an alternative to long-term care protection. This type of policy is sometimes referred to as a recovery care policy.

Let's say, like Doug, you have a family member who refuses to even consider going through underwriting other than to answer a few questions or is older than the cutoff issue age for other policy options or has limited funds. STC is an option. Once the claim is approved, it provides funding for some care needs. In some cases, it can allow the family time to consider options in case it turns out that some long-term care will be needed.

Alternately, someone considering a longer elimination period to lower the cost of a TLTC policy may use a STC policy to provide some funding while waiting for the TLTC benefits to kick in. Piggybacking the two policies, STC and TLTC, may also allow the insured to stretch out a TLTC by delaying the start of TLTC benefit payments.

Similar to long-term care insurance, once the insured qualifies and goes on claim, short-term policies typically can be used for care in the home, an assisted living facility, a nursing home, or a daycare or hospice (if there are any charges). Most short-term care insurance policies have limited benefit periods less than one full year, but some may provide a benefit for each site of care, meaning benefits may be provided for up to three years. Similar to reimbursement-type TLTC policies (discussed later), if the policyholder does not use their full daily or monthly maximum amounts, the actual benefit period stretches out, lasting longer than the elected benefit period. STC policies are guaranteed renewable, meaning the insurer cannot cancel coverage if you pay the premiums on time. Like TLTC policies, the premiums are not guaranteed and may be subject to an increase in the future for a "class" of policies.

STC is not available in every state. Some states have approved policies that offer inflation protection.

The activities of daily living (ADL) triggers for benefit eligibility for short-term care insurance generally are the same as they are for qualified long-term care coverage, meaning the policy pays for care when the insured can't perform at least two of six activities of daily living without help—eating, bathing, transferring in and out of a chair or bed, dressing, toileting and continence.

The second benefit, cognitive impairment, may differ. TLTC and other types of LTC policies may require that cognitive impairment be severe.

There are other notable differences: STC products do not have the same nonforfeiture or inflation protection options as LTC and may offer different riders, such as informal care benefits, prescription drug benefits, and/or other supplemental accident and health benefits. Also, qualified LTC contracts require that the expectation of assistance must last for a minimum of ninety days, which is not a requirement of STC policies. A third and very significant difference is, unlike TLTC, STC insurance pays in addition to Medicare.

STC is not the only limited-term option available. For younger clients or price-sensitive clients who want to go the twofers route, term insurance may present a good option.

Term insurance with an Accelerated Death Benefit Endorsement (ADBE) Rider

A term life insurance policy may be a good fit for someone who just wants to provide for their loved ones but doesn't have the desire or budget to use the policy as a financial investment. Unlike LTC, term insurance has been around a very long time. The first term life insurance company was established in Philadelphia in 1759.

Term life insurance is simple to understand. It guarantees payment of a specified death benefit to the insured's specified beneficiaries if the insured person dies during a specified term. Premiums are determined by age, health, risky activities, and term/protection period. The longer the term period, the higher the premium, because as you age, the cost of insurance increases and the more expensive years are averaged into the stated premium. Riders can also be added to term insurance. The most common include guaranteed insurability, accidental death, waiver of premium, family income benefit, child term, and return of premium riders. But the one that interests a younger member of the CPT is an accelerated death benefit endorsement (ADBE).

Term insurance with an ADBE rider can be used to offset extended and LTC risk for already stretched budgets. Individuals who may already own life insurance might want to use it to cover risks for a specific time period. The ADBE for critical, chronic, and terminal illness provides a portion of the life insurance policy's death benefit for a qualified claim, reducing or eliminating the policy's death benefit.

Doug's involvement in Step Three's CPT morphed from passive participant to active beneficiary. Additionally, it looks as if CPT participation also helps out a younger CPT generation member.

Erik texts his mom, "Is there a convenient evening for a call with you and Dad once we get the kids down? I probably need additional life insurance now that we have a second child and I am about to celebrate another birthday."

As we know, Erik and his wife are part of Generation X, born between 1965 and 1980. Unlike generations before them, they are not limited by location and rely on new technologies to conduct social and financial transactions. GenXers tend to be more attached to their profession than working for a particular company. They see entrepreneurship as a viable and challenging career option.

They grew up during the final years of the Vietnam War, Watergate, and the Reagan and Bush Senior era. They also witnessed the end of the Cold War, the expansion of globalism, the introduction of early home computers, radical changes to the media industry, and the early days of MTV. Generation X grew up with continual change and the introduction of new technologies. As a consequence, GenXers tend to be accustomed to a changing environment.[78]

Erik is a typical GenXer coveting the latest and greatest TV, technology, cars, exercise equipment, and entertainment apps. Many of his young children's toys and learning tools connect to apps and remote control devices. As the sole breadwinner of his family, Erik works hard. After accepting a promotion, he, his wife, and his children moved farther away from his family.

Jodi sets a date and time but has concerns about this new family planning dynamic. Over dinner the next evening, Jodi feels it would be wise to remind Jackson that while the CPT discussions about family and financial protection has led Erik to want to protect his own family, Jackson needs to remember not to get dictatorial or overly protective. Jackson clearly loves his children, but sometimes he forgets they are now grown adults. Their life experiences, which formed a good deal of their personalities and reactions to planning, are different from her husband's. In planning for themselves, the CPT expects Jodi or Jackson to lead the discussion. Pleased the three simple steps have reminded Erik to move forward with protecting his own family, she wonders if Jackson can turn over the reins. She also knows that Jackson is not a big fan of term insurance so that's another concern.

"Jackson, before we get involved in helping Erik with supplementing his life insurance, I think we should remember something."

"What's that?" Jackson looks up from his dinner plate.

"We are part of the baby boomer generation."

"And they are not! Got it!"

"I was just reading an article that indicated three-quarters of GenXers have higher family incomes than their parents did at the same ages, but only a third have higher wealth." [79] *Jodi pushes on before Jackson can interrupt. "In part, this is because the typical Gen Xer has six times more debt than their parents did. GenXers were hit particularly hard by falling housing values and rising unemployment rates. As a result, they lost nearly half their wealth between 2007 and 2010."* [80]

"And then there is a tremendous amount of student debt that they have to carry as well," Jackson adds, warming to the subject.

"Where I am going with this is, since this is Erik's deal, we will have to respect him in the same way he did when we were dealing with our planning. He may not want to share financial details with everyone. We come at it from a different vantage point. We will have to actively listen so we don't misunderstand or dismiss his values, lifestyle, or expectations."

"The kids did ask lots of questions as members of our Care Planning Team. They were asking questions that didn't dig too far into our personal finances or health but needed to be fleshed out in relation to the option."

Jodi reaches over and squeezes Jackson's hand. "We need to do the same for them." You can almost hear her nervous sigh of relief.

Not only will Jackson have to adjust to generational differences, but he will have to remember that he is at a very different financial stage. No matter the generation, planning starts with getting a picture of your current situation. Your priorities are likely to change as you mature; adjustments, modifications, and additions will be likely. It is essential that you continue to have a good grasp on your financial picture so that you are comfortable paying premiums currently but also in the future. As we know from planning for the grandparents and now for Jodi and Jackson, the younger you start to plan, the more options are available to you. The better your health, the less expensive the option is likely to be.

> *At the next CPT meeting, Jodi tells the group that term insurance with an ADBE is up next on the docket. She is met with some blank stares, so she quickly continues. "Some of the newer term polices come with an accelerated death benefit endorsement. An accelerated death benefit is a living benefit that allows the policyholder to access a portion of the death benefit if diagnosed with a qualifying illness."*

> *Erik asks, "Are we looking at another formula? Where's my sister?"*

Actually, this is an important point. In calculating the ADBE rider attached to a term policy, most formulas incorporate the severity of the illness, actuarial factors for past and future premiums, life expectancy, and type of coverage. Some carriers may terminate the policy if the policyholder accepts payment of the accelerated benefit.

> *If you recall, Jodi has a term policy. Her daughter thinks this is where the conversation is headed. "So, Mom, are you considering trading in your current term policy for one with an ADBE rider?"*

> *Jodi does not share Erik's request about buying term insurance with the others. Instead, Jodi addresses the topic*

as if she is considering it as one of her options. "It isn't as simple as it sounds. Life insurance pricing is age sensitive and only gets more expensive as you get older, and despite what you may think, I am not getting any younger."

That clever remark brings on all kinds of teasing from the group.

"OK, let's get serious." Jodi tries to keep a straight face as she continues. "Aside from the cost, I would also be concerned that the policy would be in force when I need it for extended or long-term care, which hopefully is a couple of decades away!"

Holding up her hand, "Don't start again!" She continues, "And there may be underwriting considerations. I don't think my health has changed since I bought my current policy, but maybe it has a little."

The CPT looks as if they are going to burst trying to restrain themselves from further teasing. Jodi holds up a warning finger.

"And finally, replacement starts a new contestability period, which means if I misstate something relevant to underwriting criteria or knowingly commit fraud, the policy is null and void."

That last remark takes the CPT over the top. Dripping with sarcasm and grinning, Erik asks, "Is that a worry, Mom? Funny you would even mention that!"

Now even Jodi is overcome with laughter.

In Jodi's case, this option is more complex, not only because of the reasons she stated—age, underwriting, conversion of the older policy, and the requirements of the new policy—but also because her need for insurance has changed. Originally, she bought term insurance to replace her income in case she died during her working years while raising young children. The death benefit would have given Jackson time to figure out a plan. Now that the children are grown, maybe considering newer term insurance with an accelerated death benefit endorsement is worth a look.

If Jodi claims and qualifies for benefits from her term insurance with an ADBE rider, and the claim reduces the death benefit and/or the policy terminates, it will serve her objective of funding some of her extended care needs.

Her other option is to keep her current term policy in place for the death benefit and apply for a hybrid policy to fund her long-term care needs. If she doesn't use the extended or long-term care rider attached to the life policy, the death benefit goes to her beneficiaries.

Erik appreciates that his mother didn't mention his request for advice. In Erik's case, since he needs additional insurance and money is tight for the young growing family, term insurance with an ADBE rider may be a good option. Although, he will need to consider converting the coverage at a later date, for the next twenty years or so, as his family grows and passes through different life stages, he double dips on coverages—life and long-term care. (He still rides his motorcycle despite his wife's protests.)

Takeaway:

It is important to create an atmosphere of trust. Discussions and questioning is an integral part of the CPT function. However, it isn't necessary to overshare personal thoughts in order for each member to benefit from reviewing planning options.

CHAPTER 34

Benefit Payments and Payout Options

I t essential to figure out how benefit payments and the payout of benefits will impact your budget, and to examine potential tax impacts with your tax advisor. There are multiple choices for premium payments:

- Monthly, quarterly, or annual premium payments from current income sources
- A lump sum or periodic payments from either pre-taxed or taxed savings or liquid investments
- Policy exchanges that may alter the payment structure
- Employer contributions or employee payroll deductions

Equally important is to understand the benefit payout designs. Some contracts only offer indemnity payouts while others offer reimbursement or cash indemnity payouts or a disability model with a fixed benefit and trigger requirement. The most common are indemnity or reimbursement models.[81]

Reimbursement vs. Cash Indemnity Payout of Benefits

	Reimbursement	Cash Indemnity
Eligibility Requirements	The insured is certified as chronically ill, has a plan of care and satisfied the elimination period	The insured is certified as chronically ill, has a plan of care and satisfied the elimination period
Monthly LTC Benefit	Only expenses incurred on qualified services are reimbursed, not to exceed the monthly maximum	Up to 100% of the monthly maximum is paid as a cash benefit. The stated dollar amount of the per diem limitation (guaranteed tax free, benefit, or reimbursed amount) is $400 for tax year 2021.
Monthly Bill & Receipts	Required	Not required
Informal Care	Limited or no coverage	Yes
Restrictions on Use of Benefits	Limited to qualified LTC expenses incurred as defined in the contract	None

Courtesy LTCI Partners, LLC http://www.ltcipartners.com Steve Cain, steve.cain@ltcipartners.com (608) 283-6600

The upside of a reimbursement method is that once you are approved for benefits, you receive a benefit equal to the total cost of qualified services, up to the policy's predetermined maximum. With reimbursements, since only the expenses incurred each month are paid out of the maximum benefit pool of money available from the contract, benefit cost coverage may stretch out over a longer period. Since these costs are tied to the actual cost of benefits, there is no tax implications for monies received.

The downside of the reimbursement method is that if the care expenses exceed the monthly benefit, there could be out-of-pocket costs. However, if you decide to buy a policy that funds only a portion of anticipated costs, that may translate into a smaller and more affordable policy premium. In that case, your financial plan should include provisions for you to personally fund the potential balance yourself.

With the indemnity method, as a result of monthly payments of a fixed amount, regardless of incurred care costs, the pool of money may be exhausted more quickly and there may be a tax implication.

What do these two options look like in action? The process for reimbursement is as follows: You incur expenses, collect and submit receipts, then the carrier reviews and approves the receipts before issuing payment. Many insurers will arrange for direct payments to the facility or care provider.

The indemnity insurance method pays a policyholder a fixed amount of cash when you experience a qualified covered event, meet the policy's requirements, and are approved for benefits. The upside of this method is that once you qualify for benefits, you are virtually on your own to pay medical and nonmedical expenses. You don't need to offer proof to the insurer that the benefit spending is being used for long-term care or chronic condition needs. As so often happens in life, this upside comes with a caveat. If the benefit payments exceed the greater of the established IRS per diem annual limit, or to state it in plain English, the actual qualified long-term care incurred expenses are less than the amount of money you receive, the difference becomes taxable as income. So, while you may not have to provide proof to the insurer that the benefits were used for the payment of long-term care expenses, you may want to keep a record of disbursements in case you need to provide the IRS with proof of expenditures, which may be as simple as a copy of payments made to a facility. If the amount exceeds the IRS set limit of the annual per diem (daily) dollar amount but the amount is totally allocated to the reimbursement of long-term care expenses, then there is no taxation issue.

Insurance companies that pay long-term care insurance benefits are required by the Internal Revenue Service (IRS) to provide claimants with a 1099-LTC."[82]

Having a pretty firm handle on premium and benefit payment methods, the CPT is ready to move on to selecting options to discuss with professionals. Advisement is not only smart but helps avoid unknown pitfalls and may influence your final selection.

Takeaway:

How premium payments and benefit payout methods align with your projected short- and long-term budget represents another important planning consideration.

CHAPTER 35

Figuring Out Your Financial Assets and Obligations

Like so many of us, life is busy, and we often do not readily have an overall picture of our financial assets and obligations. To help a young family (or any individual/family/partners) understand what they can currently afford and to plan for future affordability in selecting an option, a question-and-answer session may be helpful. Whether planning on your own, as a CPT member, or meeting with an agent or advisor, this exercise may reveal priorities and issues.

Answering questions/topics that apply to you should help you create a document or fill in an online budget tool to kickstart your path to a more solid understanding of your financial picture.

- Do you have a monthly budget? Do you usually stick to it?
- What kind of debt do you have?
  - Credit cards?

- Auto loans?
- Student loans?
- Do you own a home or rent?
  - Mortgage?
  - Second mortgage?
  - Lines of credit?
- Do you use layaway plans or periodic payment plans?
- Do you see yourself staying in your current residence?
  - Are you planning to age in place?
  - Are you planning to start a family or do you have a growing family?
  - Will your children go to a neighborhood school or elsewhere?
  - Are you responsible for the welfare or well-being of someone else?
- Will you want to earn a degree or professional designation? What is its estimated cost?
- What does your current savings plan look like?
- Do you pay someone to handle your savings and investments?
- Do you expect to receive an inheritance (money, property, jewelry, bitcoin, etc.)?
- Do you know if you are listed as a beneficiary of anyone's life insurance or qualified savings plans (such as a 401(k) or IRA)?
- Will you inherit a family business? Is it a profitable business?
- Is your health-care coverage tied to employment?
  - Are premiums deducted out of your paycheck?
  - Do you purchase other supplemental benefits that are deducted from your paycheck?
- How do you pay for insurance coverage?
- What types of insurance do you have?
  - Homeowners or renters
  - Life insurance (with or without riders?)
    o Permanent or Term?

- Annuity (with or without riders?)
- Auto, motorcycle, or boat insurance
- Do you usually reach your health-care plan's deductible?
- Are prescription drug costs totally covered?
- Do you have vision, dental, or hearing plan payments?
- Do you have any reoccurring payments through employment or on your own?
- Do you have an FSA or HSA account?
- Do you or another family member/partner access any government-sponsored benefits?
- Do you contribute to any charities (such as a school alma mater)?
- Does your spouse/partner plan to go to work full-time? If yes, indicate number of years or planned date of retirement.
- Would you be willing to move if either of you were offered an out-of-state job?
- Does your employer offer a match for 401(k) contributions? Are there any outstanding loans?
- Do you have an employer-sponsored savings plan that is still with a previous employer or one that is rolled over into an IRA?
- Do you or your spouse/partner have another savings vehicle, like an IRA or 401(k)?
- Are you retired or plan to soon retire? Will you relocate after retirement?
- Other financially important information.

There are side benefits to this exercise. Thanks to reviewing the list with his wife, among other things, Erik is reminded that he left his 401(k) at a previous employer. According to the latest white paper by Capitalize Research, *The True Cost of Forgotten 401(k) Accounts (2021)*, they estimate that there are 24.3 million forgotten 401(k)s holding $1.35 trillion in assets, as of May 2021. Importantly, an additional 2.8 million accounts are left-behind by job changers each year, though some will eventually be reclaimed or liquidated. In aggregate, savers could be missing out on a combined $116 billion in additional retirement savings each year by leaving behind 401(k) accounts.[83]

Erik is chatting with his sister. They are discussing the new home he bought when he moved his family to a new town for a new job. "Speaking of moving, I was reviewing the list of questions. It included questions about 401(k)s. Honestly, I have been so busy that I haven't even given it any thought. I guess I should add it to my to-do list before I forget about it."

"I get it," says Nicole. "You need to focus on the present and that's a lot! But saving is part of a good plan. Let me pitch in. I'll arrange a call for you and my advisor. He can at least let you know what your options are. Then, you can decide what works best for you and yours. At least your investments and savings should grow while you are earning and figuring out family protections."

Nicole's advisor texts Erik and they arrange a call. "Hello, Erik. My name is Joe.[84] Your sister let me know that you have some questions about a 401(k) that you left at your previous employment when you changed jobs. First, let me start by complimenting you for contributing to your 401(k) plan.

My understanding is that you and your wife are now using an online tool to keep yourselves up to date on where you're spending money and what will be set aside for savings. That is a great first step in financial preparedness. I also understand that the immediate issue that you want to discuss is if you should move your 401(k) plan to an IRA account."

"Here is how I suggest we approach this. We'll review the underlying funds expense ratio plus the plan sponsor fees to determine if it's more beneficial to rollover a 401(k) to an IRA or to keep the 401(k) with your previous employer."

"Are the funds just as safe if held in my own IRA instead of in an employer's plan?"

"The money held in your employer's ERISA-qualified 401(k) retirement plan is protected by the Employee Retirement Income Security Act of 1974 from claims by creditors but not from the IRS, which I am sure doesn't surprise you."

"Not really! Do you lose that protection when you roll the money into an IRA account?"

"Any amount rolled over from a qualified plan to an IRA is protected from creditors under federal bankruptcy law. Outside of that, protection from creditors is based on state law."

"What's the advantage of rolling it over?"

"Leaving a 401(k) plan with your previous employer means you may be limited to their funds menu if the plan does not allow the option of a self-directed brokerage account within the company's 401(k) plan. If you rollover the funds to an IRA, your investment choices would be unlimited. I sent you a text with a link to some reading material on the topic.[85] While the IRA may provide you with a wider range of investment options, and likely may be less expensive, it does mean giving up some of the

*benefits of a 401(k), depending on the plan documents,
like hardship withdrawals and loan provisions. Since I
am unable to offer tax or legal advice, I must insist that
you consult your tax advisor as well."*

*"Yup, as a member of my grandparents' and parents' Care
Planning Teams, I think I have that advice down pat!"*

*Amused but not fully understanding Erik's remark, Joe
simply replies, "Good!" Moving on, he becomes more
serious, "In order to recommend the proper investment
plan, I would likely need to take you through the process
I use in order to confirm your investment goals."*

*"Sounds good. Let's get a date on the calendar now so
I don't get so involved in something else that I postpone
this. I know it is just as important to pay attention to
savings and investments as it is to earn more money
through promotions!"*

*Joe meets with Erik and his wife to make sure they can
articulate and understand their investment goals and
risk tolerance before he makes a recommendation. "Based
on you feeling comfortable with an aggressive investment
allocation, your young age in proximity to retirement/
projected need for the funds, and your goals, we reviewed
an allocation for your IRA that is heavily weighted toward equities. We went through many details, including
fees and expenses. I feel you understand the risks inherent
in such an allocation. Now, we can move forward."*

*"Joe, thanks for carefully explaining the pros and cons of
moving the 401(k) account from my previous employer.
I feel confident, and my CPA agrees, that the benefits*

of moving that 401(k) account to an IRA outweigh the benefits of leaving the funds with my previous employer."

"Good to hear. I will send you the proper paperwork to complete, an IRA application and a rollover request to DocuSign. I will also send you a calendar invitation for a final review and to answer any other investment questions you may have. I look forward to working with you over the years."

Takeaway:

Topics and conversations that may seem unrelated to extended or long-term care planning can be a catalyst to overall improved financial family wellness planning, for younger generations as well as those closer to retirement.

CHAPTER 36

Trading in Current Coverage for Coverage with a Rider

Getting the best possible financial outcome from the assets and insurance contracts that you already own is simply smart. Refreshing your overall financial picture by revisiting budget and spending questions is also smart. The more information you have, the easier it is to select extended and long-term care options that preserve your good efforts.

While Erik and his mother, Jodi, may each consider a term policy with a rider but for different reasons, Jackson always believed in owning permanent insurance. He listed a whole life insurance policy that has built up a good deal of cash in his summary document. He could borrow against the cash value if he needed funds for long-term care. However, if he pulls money out to pay for care, the distribution, above the premiums paid into the policy, would be taxable.

An option to avoid paying taxes on the growth and cover his need for funding long-term care expenses is a Section 1035 exchange. A

1035 exchange is a provision in the IRS code allowing for a tax-free transfer of an existing annuity contract, life insurance policy, long-term care product, or endowment for another one of like kind.

If Jackson opts to do a 1035 exchange of his current policy for a life insurance policy with a long-term care rider, his primary benefit would be that the significant cash buildup in his current policy could become a tax-free distribution if he qualifies, his claim is approved, and he uses the funds to pay for extended or long-term care.

However, there are also reasons why exchanging his existing policy for a new one may be challenging. There could be underwriting criteria that Jackson would have to meet, fees, including commissions, a surrender charge, other expenses, higher pricing due to the change in his age or health, a new contestability period during which the insurance company could challenge a death claim based on a material misstatement on the application. For a policy with an outstanding loan, there could also be a tax implication unless the loan is paid back before the exchange takes place.[86]

If Jackson wants to place his new policy with a different carrier from his current insurer, the existing contract must be transferred directly to the new insurance carrier. The new carrier would surrender the existing contract and issue a new one.[87]

Anyone considering a 1035 exchange should consult with their CPA or tax advisor since the owner is required to submit a 1099-R form to the IRS unless the new life insurance policy is held by the same company from which the funds are being transferred. It would be terrible to move forward with an exchange and create a tax liability.

So much of planning for current and future health-care costs revolves around education, preparation, and professional advice. Sometimes friends also can be a good resource for moving things forward. Jodi hesitated to share the burden of caregiving with her own family. At first, she doesn't do much better with a friend in need.

Jodi meets a longtime friend for coffee. She notices that her friend looks worn out. She knows her friend's story.

Her friend's parents were unprepared for a long-term care event. It just tore their family apart. She felt guilty that, at the time, she was not more helpful. It's such a tough subject to address. Although her own family achieved peace of mind by using the three simple steps, had the Care Guide ready for the emergency, snapped into action using the Care Squad assignments, and uncovered noninsurance solutions for funding her parents' care in their home, Jodi just listened quietly but didn't offer her friend any advice. She didn't want to sound like a know-it-all, or worse, judgmental.

Noticing how more relaxed and healthier Jodi looks, her friend asks, "How did you handle being the parent to your parents?"

"We discovered a tool to start the conversation without actually lecturing anyone or making someone feel as if they are a problem to be handled. It's just three simple steps. I suggest you try it. Makes you feel saner."

Her friend, miserable, is desperate. "I will try it. I'll talk to my brother about it. Somehow, he seems to think that help and funding is just falling out of the sky."

"You sound angry," Jodi responds honestly. "Maybe consider that he simply may not know about the possibility of a more workable option?"

Her friend, to Jodi's surprise, considers the possibility, but then flatly states, "Well, we'll see if he, or for that matter his wife, will consider discussing options. Maybe letting them know about the three simple steps will let them see possible approaches or alternatives." Her friend's tone reveals some bitterness, "Even if we only do a couple of the steps, maybe I will feel more in control and ready to seek out some advice. After all, we still have our aging father to worry about. I'm not at all sure our relationship will survive another difficult, stressful situation."

"Don't feel bad. I tried to do it all on my own too. Thank goodness my kids pointed out what it was doing to me and generations above and beneath me. After reviewing various options, we consulted with several specialists, and to everyone's relief, we got things planned out."

Conceding the relationship with her friend's brother and his wife is already strained, Jodi quickly adds, "You may need to seek out an advisor to run through a list of options if family tensions are running too high. That way, it is a third party carving a path to sanity. We were lucky that each of our CPT members wanted to participate and contribute."

"Your CPT? What's that?"

Jodi air hugs her friend, "Go over the three simple steps and you'll see."

Takeaway:

It can be challenging for friends or family to work together once care needs surface, become demanding, and create family tension. Instead of offering details, maybe suggest a direction to alleviate a worsening situation, such as the three simple steps, or engage an advisor or elder-care attorney as a facilitator.

CHAPTER 37

When to Consider Professional Advisement

Nowadays, so many of us turn to friends for advice and recommendations. In order to best utilize good advice and keep the planning simple, understandable, flexible, and affordable, preparation is key. Using the three simple steps to create a helpful environment, delineate roles, unearth options, and formulate questions aids friends and multiple family generations in planning and is useful for effectively guiding professionals in understanding priorities and possibilities.

As we saw, not every personal or financial detail is shared with either of the Jones family Care Planning Teams; not every detail needs be shared. A basic grasp of the general social, familial, financial, psychological, health, and well-being picture works. My three simple steps is an inclusive but not an invasive approach.

- Step One's Care Guide helps organize essential health and legal documentation information.
- Step Two's Care Squad organizes individuals into an action ready unit.
- Step Three's Care Planning Team investigates options for taking care of extended or long-term care needs, including a basic understanding of eligibility and financial feasibility.

Each generation can employ the three simple steps according to their own individuality, timeline, needs, and view of the world. When seeking advice, most families will interact with several categories of advisors who all serve different roles. Depending on your particular situation, you may call on a financial advisor, insurance agent, business tax consultant, CPA, investment advisor, age-in-place expert, eldercare attorney, legal counsel, Medicare/Medicaid specialist, reverse mortgage specialist, and so on.

Unlike the GenXer and Millennial children in the family who may seek recommendations from friends or social media, Jodi and Jackson's generational orientation led them to a more formal method of selecting an advisor. Let's hear them discuss how they checked out the professional credentials and reputation of their advisor.

> Jodi says, "We know being an educated consumer is strategic for family cohesiveness and helpful when seeking advice. Once Jackson and I select the options or product types we want to further investigate, we'll make a list of our questions. Ethical advisors and agents, like ours, want clients to purchase the right product. The entire process is now easier since we can share pertinent thoughts and ask informed questions as a result of the three simple steps."

> "Agree, Mom." After a moment, Nicole continues, "Not only does Step Three speed up the selection process, but

later you won't be unsure of what exactly you bought and neither will your children when you aren't there to explain your reasons for purchasing a product. But the challenge is, how do you select the right advisor before you start sharing your personal information?"

Jodi was very careful when she and her dad, James, selected an advisor. Now she and Jackson work with that same advisor. She knew that other members of the family would probably ask her for a recommendation. However, as parents, she and Jackson advised Erik and Nicole to interview several candidates so the advisor would align with their generational orientation as well as personal objectives.

Nicole asks, "What criteria did you look for in an advisor?" Jodi isn't surprised by Nicole's follow-up question. Erik teases her all the time about being a detail junkie.

Nicole answers her own question. "I know what I did when I selected my investment advisor, but insurance and other options are not in his wheelhouse. I am sure he can recommend someone. Otherwise, I can check with the Division of Insurance State Licensing Bureau to see if an agent or advisor has any violations or disciplinary actions against them. Also, the fee structure or commission schedule should be easy to understand and transparent, so I feel comfortable that I can afford to pay for the services. And speaking of services, I guess I should first decide what services I need."

Erik suggests, "Well, that really depends on what you want out of the relationship, doesn't it, Nicole?"

"Yeah, true. For me, one of the basic requirements was that they focused on building a long-lasting relationship

and not just a quick sale. I also need them to translate the complicated aspects of insurance into simpler explanations a non-industry person can understand."

"You know, Nicole," her brother offers, "we should also look for evidence that they adhere to established ethical practices and invest in themselves by accessing updated information and industry developments. I would check to see if they are involved in speaking or writing, or belong to a professional association."

"Actually," Jodi jumps in to explain why it was important when she evaluated her advisor. "NAIFA has several specialty centers. One of them is the Limited and Extended Care Planning Center."[88]

Jackson, who had left the room for a couple of minutes, walks back in. Unlike Jodi, who is an active listener, letting her children share thoughts and ideas, Jackson is more of the take-charge type. Jumping back onscreen, he says, "I caught the tail end of that conversation. Our advisor is a CLTC, which means she has earned a Certification in Long-term Care.[89] We feel it's important to work with a professional who understands the complexity of what it means to effectively plan. They don't just sell product. Our advisor has invested in additional training and meets regular continuing education requirements. She also has several other designations and certifications from the American College of Financial Services. She is a CLU, a ChFC, and a CASL. She says it helps her manage difficult conversations and focus on developing professional and personalized plans."

"Before this call, Mom and I sat down to eliminate some extended and long-term care options, like we did with your grandparents. We saw no point in talking with our advisor about options that don't work with what we want to achieve, don't fit with our budget, or for which we won't qualify. Once we have a sense of what we want, we will consult with our advisor and ask our tax guy's opinion. They may point something out to change our direction, but they will have gained an understanding of our thinking on the subject."

"Are there any options that you already discussed or discarded?" Not wanting to appear pushy, Nicole quickly adds, *"Just curious!"*

"Well, yeah, there are. For example, we are concerned about traditional long-term care premium rate increases."

Jodi attempts to turn the discussion away from particular options until she is more comfortable with their selections. *"Dad has a subscription to the* Wall Street Journal. *In a recent article, the financial columnist, Glenn Ruffenach, discusses the importance of planning for long-term care and points to the Shopper's Guide[90] as a valuable resource. Ruffenach also agrees that 'your best first step is not to shop for a carrier or policy. Rather, it's to shop for a knowledgeable, independent agent.'"*

"We accessed a copy of our state's Shopper's Guide online and then called our advisor." Continuing to miss his wife's detour, he continues, *"We will consider, along with other details, the company's rating and their rate increase history. If that turns out to be a deal breaker for us, we will look at a hybrid contract, which hopefully has some*

meaningful guarantees. We need our agent to do that homework for us, but we are armed with questions so she understands our priorities."

Takeaway:

Personalizing information and selecting a qualified advisor is important to a good working relationship. Seeking advisement is smart and helps avoid unknown pitfalls that may influence a final selection.

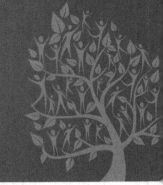

CHAPTER 38

On Becoming an Educated Consumer

Jackson and Jodi are ready to narrow down their choices so they can engage their advisory team. They have almost completed the three simple steps.

As better-educated consumers, with a grasp of current budget and future monetary obligations (money going out), how they want to receive benefit payments (money coming in), health underwriting considerations, and personal opinions about product and service preferences in hand, they are ready to move forward!

Narrowing Down Options to the Best Fit

Jodi and Jackson share an insurance cheat sheet[91] to review several of their options.

Long-Term Care Insurance	Asset Based Hybrid	Life Insurance	Fixed or Indexed Annuities	Self Funded
Protect your assets from an extended health care event	Protect your assets and retirement savings from an extended health care event while retaining maximum flexibility	Maximize your death benfit while retaining moderate flexibility	Long-term care options late in life with potential health concern	Access to money now

PROS:

Long-Term Care Insurance	Asset Based Hybrid	Life Insurance	Fixed or Indexed Annuities	Self Funded
- Inflation Protecation - Care Coordination "Concierge Healthcare" Benefit - Maximizes long-term care insurance leverage while minimizing premium committment - Tax deductibile for business owners - HSAs	- Standardized benfit trigger - 1035 exchanges - Tax advantages - Maximizes flexibility and provides a substantial benefit for a long-term care insurance event - Flexibile payment options - Return of premium - Guaranteed premiums - Life insurance and LTC Benefits	- Largest death benefits - Relitively low premium cost for rider - Better suited to pay for benefits on a monthly basis, if needed	- Limited or no medical underwriting - 1035 exchange tax advantage could turn tax-deferred growth to tax-free LTC payments	- Zero up-front costs while retaining liquidity

CONS:

Long-Term Care Insurance	Asset Based Hybrid	Life Insurance	Fixed or Indexed Annuities	Self Funded
- Premiums not guaranteed - "Use it or lose it" premium (no chase value or return of premium	- Opportunity cost (if single premium option is selected) - Not the same tax advntages for business owners	- If LTC is needed, reduction of death benefit - No return of premium - Benefit triggers not standardized - Benefits determined at claim time - No inflation protection	- Limited or no inflation protection - Typically no care coordination - No tax advantages for business owners	- Not a healthcare plan - No care coodination benefit - Tax timing consequences

Courtesy LTCI Partners, LLC http://www.ltcipartners.com Steve Cain, steve.cain@ltcipartners.com (608) 283-6600

Jodi starts off the review. "*Somewhat like what your grandparents did before sharing with their entire Care Planning Team, we narrowed down our choices. We worked with our broker who offered us a chart to help the three of us move through and focus on options that best fit our objectives and budget.*"

"*Starting from the right side of the chart, here are our thoughts.*"

"*As for self-funding, if you recall, we used a cost-of-care website to estimate future costs ten or fifteen years into the future. We concluded that we do not want to keep a large portion of our investment portfolio locked up and dedicated to the possibility of one or both of us needing extended care. Worse, we worry that even a large sum may be quickly depleted, leaving the other person in a bad situation."*

Jackson takes over, "We feel that underwriting is not an issue for either of us. We are still young enough to build some equity in a product, and we like the deferred taxation aspect of deferred annuities. Our broker mentioned that there is one insurer that offers a discount for two insureds who buy a policy together and a death benefit that pays heirs when the surviving spouse dies if the long-term care benefits used up the funds."

"We want to discuss the 1035 exchange with our CPA. I want to see about loaning the cash value built up in my whole life insurance policy versus possibly doing a 1035 exchange so the significant cash buildup in my policy could become a tax-free distribution if I qualify to use the funds to pay for extended or long-term care. That being said, we discussed my meeting underwriting criteria, fees, including commissions, a surrender charge, other expenses, higher pricing due to any changes in my age or health, and a new contestability period. We'll consult with our agent since that will take some analyzing!"

Jodi adds, "We're also interested in life insurance hybrids and traditional long-term care insurance policies. Alternately, I'm interested in a term policy with an ADBE."

Jackson and Jodi look at each other in agreement. Jackson wraps up, "We'll call the broker and ask for some quotes and dig into the details. We'll share the quotes and advice so you completely understand what we choose, why

*we select it, and our financial commitment to taking this
potential family burden off the table."*

Jodi and Jackson intend to do the work to create real peace of
mind by knowing they worked on the best plan for themselves and the
generations that follow them. Although not too many personal health
or financial details were shared, when the time comes and one or both
of them require any level of care, the entire family will not only know
what's in place, but importantly, they will know how to help. They will
simply use the first two of the three simple steps.

> *Once final selections are made and the policies are in
> place, Jodi arranges a final CPT call and sends a bottle
> of celebratory wine to each household. On the next call,
> they all toast to the success and peace of mind that comes
> with the completion of the three simple steps.*
>
> *Jackson raises his glass. "Here's to not having our retire-
> ment destroyed by unforeseen costs or worrying about
> becoming a burden to each other or to any of you!"*
>
> *Jodi, looking like a different person from when they first
> started going through the three simple steps with her
> parents, adds, "And we gave each other fitness watches
> as an anniversary gift and an exercise bike as a bonus
> for completing the three simple steps! Cheers, everyone!*

Takeaway:

The only plan you are destined to have is the one you decide to create.

CONCLUDING
THOUGHTS AND
ENCOURAGEMENT

Thank you for joining me and the Jones family as they tackled the daunting issue of starting the conversation and following the three simple steps to a successful conclusion. For most of us, the tricky part is that life doesn't stop while you're caught up in caring and juggling. Family life, however you define your family, is dynamic and ever changing.

If you are not yet caught in the sandwich generation, like Jodi, with parents, siblings, or grandparents on the brink of an emergency, don't wait until it's too late! Without realizing it, you may slowly assume the role of the on-site, on-call, or long-distance caregiver who is untrained, unprepared, and eventually unable to manage all that is expected of you.

For many of us, the idea of a role reversal with someone you love is scary. The role of a family caregiver often requires that you give up more than just your lifestyle. You may put your own future financial stability at risk.

The primary objective of the three simple steps is to offer an easy-to-follow, easily adaptable process. But you must start! My three simple steps offer you three different approaches to get started and not tear you or your family physically, psychologically, or financially apart.

First, the advantages of having a Care Guide that is as complete as possible is undeniable. It's a *caring* conversation. As we saw, different generations of the Jones family approached it according to their generational orientation. From writing it out, sealing a Care Guide in an envelope to be kept in a cache or entrusted to a family member or friend, to electronically storing it and giving access as needed, do what suits you best. Inspiration usually comes with experience. Hopefully, identifying with the grandparents' event provided you with the motivation.

What about Step Two? Maybe you prefer to start the *what if* conversation. What if your child gets hurt at school? What if you are unprepared, leading to bitterness and anger? What if your family is being torn apart because you didn't know how to invite or prepare anyone to divide care chores? When Jackson and Jodi form their Care Squad, they consider schedules, availability, and practicalities. Explore the idea of a positive, well-orchestrated situation before it becomes stressful and chaotic.

Or, third, maybe you start with the *discovery* conversation. Be inclusive in forming your team. Remember when someone was left out or excluded in high school, a team, or a group? It didn't feel good. It created an aura of friction. Work together like the Jones family, exploring options while still respecting privacy. Give voice to your personal wishes and dig into the details of possible options. Options discussed in this book may change, and others will be introduced as time goes by. If you don't control your own destiny, someone else will. A lack of actionable planning can quickly translate into unwanted and unintended serious negative consequences. Work toward an option that will save you and yours from financial distress, to say nothing of emotional misery. Seek professional guidance to iron out the good, the bad, and the ugly.

The three simple steps cut through the clutter. Keep it simple. Be intentional about the challenges you face. Avoid counterproductive family stress or conflict that can tear your family apart. Instead, open a *discovery* conversation and create an actionable plan. Many of the options that you discovered with the Jones family are not tied to costly expenditures. When you are ready to seek advisement from an agent, advisor, specialist, attorney, eldercare specialist, or other professional, you are three steps ahead.

Caring involves a continuum of tiny and sometimes major changes and adjustments. It is an emotional journey but one that you can handle with a plan in place. Use whichever of the three simple steps works for you, in whatever order; use whatever type or size of CPT or support system you need. Please, just get started! The three simple steps will get you to where you need to be—personally and financially prepared, and generationally at peace. Plan. Don't panic!

> "Nothing in life is to be feared.
> It is only to be understood."
> (Marie Curie)

GLOSSARY

1035 exchange: A 1035 exchange is a provision in the Internal Revenue Service (IRS) code allowing for a tax-free transfer of an existing annuity contract, life insurance policy, long-term care product, or endowment for another one of like kind. To qualify for a Section 1035 exchange, the contract or policy owner must also meet certain other requirements.

401(K) plan: A 401(k) plan is popularly known as an employer-sponsored retirement plan to which certain eligible employees based on preset criteria can make tax-deferred contributions from their salary or wages. The employee contribution is pre-tax.

accelerated death benefit endorsement rider: this rider provides pre-payment of a portion of the death benefit when proof that an insured has been certified as a terminally ill individual and the conditions described in this rider are met, allowing the insured to use the benefit while the insured is still living.

accelerated death benefit rider: An accelerated death benefit (ADB) allows a life insurance policy owner to receive a portion of their death benefit from their insurance company in advance of their death.

accidental death benefit rider: This is a provision in a life insurance policy that can provide an additional payment if your death occurs as the result of an accident, often double the amount of money.

activities of daily living (ADL): The activities of daily living are classified into basic ADLs and instrumental activities of daily living (IADLs). The ADLs basically relate to physical skills or needs, including personal hygiene or grooming. In long-term care, they usually include transferring, dressing, toileting, continence, bathing, dressing, and eating. The ADLs for short-term care may include medication management, personal hygiene, eating, toileting, transferring, body care, bathing, ambulation/mobility, dressing, and cognitive impairment.

IADLs are skills we need in order to live independently, such as using the telephone, shopping, preparing meals, housekeeping, using transportation, taking medications, and managing finances.

advance directives: Advance directives generally fall into three categories: living will, power of attorney, and health-care proxy. These directives pertain to treatment preferences and the designation of a surrogate decision maker in the event that a person should become unable to make medical decisions on their own behalf.

annuitization phase: The annuitization phase, also known as the annuity phase, is the period when the annuitant starts to receive payments from the annuity. This period comes after the accumulation phase, which is when the money is invested in the annuity.

annuity: An annuity is a contract between you and an insurance company or similar financial institution under which, in exchange for a lump sum or ongoing premium payments, the insurance company agrees to make regular payments for either the rest of your life or for a predetermined number of years.

asset: An asset is a resource with economic value that an individual or corporation owns or controls with the expectation that it will provide a future benefit. Insurance products may use an asset in an underlying policy structure.

assisted living facility: Assisted living facilities are referred to as ALFs in the senior living industry. Assisted living facilities may provide a homelike atmosphere. Services vary depending on a resident's needs. Services may include meals, cleaning, shopping for groceries, laundry, and transportation. Newer ALFs may also be referred to as independent living arrangements. They may be simply any housing arrangement designed exclusively for older adults, generally those aged fifty-five or over. Often, recreational centers or clubhouses are available on site to give you the opportunity to connect with peers and participate in community activities. They may also offer facilities such as a swimming pool, fitness center, tennis courts, even a golf course or other clubs and interest groups. Other services offered may include on-site spas, beauty and barber salons, daily meals, and basic housekeeping and laundry services.

benefit amount, or pool of money: The benefit amount in a contract is calculated by multiplying your daily benefit amount by the number of days in your benefit period. For example, a $200 daily benefit x 365 days x 3-year benefit period = a pool of money of $219,000.

benefit triggers: Benefit triggers are the criteria that an insurance company will use to determine if you are eligible for benefits.

care coordination: Care coordination is the deliberate organization of patient care activities between two or more participants involved in a patient's care to facilitate the appropriate delivery of health-care services. Ideally, it involves collaboration between all members of a care team, no matter their specialty, role, or location.

cash value life insurance: Cash value life insurance is a type of permanent *life insurance* that includes an investment feature. *Cash value* is the portion of your policy that earns interest.

children's term rider: A children's term rider is an optional form of life insurance coverage available for purchase in addition to primary life insurance coverage.

chronic illness: A chronic illness can generally be defined as a condition with no medical cure that may last for years.

chronological age: Chronological age is your actual age based on your birth certificate.

cognitive impairment: Cognitive impairment is when a person has trouble remembering, learning new things, concentrating, or making decisions that affect their everyday life.

continuing care retirement community (CCRC): Continuing care retirement communities are multilevel care facilities that combine residential accommodations with health services for older adults. CCRCs allow residents to age in place since residents can move within levels of care while staying in the same community.

CPA: A certified public accountant (CPA) is a designation given by the American Institute of Certified Public Accountants (AICPA) to individuals who pass the Uniform CPA Examination and meet the education and experience requirements.

deferred annuities: Deferred annuities are purchased with either a single sum or flexible contributions over time and provide income payments to the annuitant that begins at some future date.

deferred growth: Tax-deferred growth is investment growth that's not subject to taxes immediately but is instead taxed at a later date.

Deficit Reduction Act (DRA) of 2005: The DRA tightens asset transfer rules to reduce the incidence of individuals transferring a substantial amount of their money and other assets to relatives in order to be eligible for long-term care services under Medicaid. The DRA also authorized expansion of the Long-Term Care Partnership Program.

defined benefit plans: A defined benefit plan, commonly referred to as a pension, is a retirement account with the benefit set up by the employer. It may be paid out as a monthly or annual payment in retirement, based on the employee's tenure and salary. Employees are not expected to contribute to the plan, and they do not have individual accounts.

defined contribution plans: The contribution is a designated amount from the employee, who has a personal account within the plan and chooses investments for it. The employee owns the account and, within plan rules, can withdraw or transfer the fund.

discounted chronic illness riders: Discounted chronic illness riders are only underwritten for the life insurance component of the policy. The applicant may have to choose if they want the rider, or it may just be included if the base policy is issued at a certain underwriting class to qualify for the rider. Although there is no charge for the chronic illness rider, it's not really free. If the chronic illness rider is activated, then a portion of the death benefit is accelerated to provide chronic illness benefits. The acceleration benefit amount is discounted to pay for the rider using a formula that comprises many factors.

dollar-for-dollar chronic illness riders: Dollar-for-dollar chronic illness riders are usually fully underwritten for both the death benefit and chronic illness. There is an explicit charge for the chronic illness rider. When the accelerated death benefit (ADB) is paid out, there is a dollar-for-dollar reduction in the face amount and a pro rata reduction in the cash value based on the percentage of the face amount that was accelerated. The full amount of the death benefit may be paid either as chronic illness benefits, a death benefit, or a combination of both.

do-not-resuscitate (DNR) order: A do-not-resuscitate order is a medical order written by a doctor. It instructs health-care providers not to do cardiopulmonary resuscitation (CPR) if a patient's breathing stops or if the patient's heart stops beating.

elder law attorney: An elder law attorney is an advocate for the elderly and their loved ones. Most elder law attorneys handle a wide range of legal matters affecting an older or disabled person, including issues related to health care, long-term care planning, guardianship, retirement, social security, Medicare/Medicaid, elder abuse, financial scams and other important matters.

elimination period: Simply stated, an elimination period is like a health insurance deductible. It's the number of days you pay for care before the policy pays.

extension of benefits (EOB) rider: An EOB rider is also referred to as a living benefit, which allows policyholders to access death benefits from their insurance policy under certain conditions while they are alive.

family caregiver: A family caregiver can be anyone who's not getting paid to help others who cannot manage daily tasks independently. Caregivers can be friends, partners, relatives, or neighbors, and the type of care they provide varies dramatically.

family income benefit rider: A family income benefit rider provides monthly income to a family after the insured's death, in addition to the lump-sum payout from a life insurance policy.

FICA taxes: The Federal Insurance Contributions Act (FICA) is a US law that mandates a payroll tax on the paychecks of employees, as well as contributions from employers, to fund the Social Security and Medicare programs. For self-employed persons, there is an equivalent law called the Self-Employed Contributions Act (SECA).

fixed annuity: Fixed annuity contracts guarantee a minimum credited interest.

fixed deferred annuity: In fixed deferred annuity contracts, the insurer credits a fixed interest rate to contributions in the accumulation phase and pays a fixed income payment in the annuitization phase.

flexible care cash amendment: A flexible care cash amendment provides clients additional benefit flexibility with access to receipt-free cash to help cover informal care needs at home, including an opportunity for a spouse to provide the care.

flexible savings account (FSA): In a flexible savings account, also known as a flexible spending arrangement, individuals contribute money into a special account and then use it to pay for certain out-of-pocket health-care costs. Employers may make contributions to FSA accounts but are not required to.

full retirement age (FRA): Full retirement age, also known as normal retirement age, is the age at which people can receive full retirement benefits upon leaving the workforce.

guaranteed insurability (GI) riders: Guaranteed insurability riders are available on certain life insurance policies and allows individuals to purchase additional insurance at specific dates in the future (subject to minimums and maximums) without having to go through an exam or answer health questions.

Health Insurance Portability and Accountability Act (HIPAA): HIPAA is a federal law that requires the creation of national standards to protect sensitive patient health information from being disclosed without the patient's consent or knowledge.[92] HIPAA also provides that a contract issued before January 1, 1997, is treated as a qualified long-term care insurance contract if the contract met state requirements for such a contract at the time it was issued. The notice sets forth rules for determining the issue date of both individual and group contracts.

health savings account (HSA): HSAs are tax-advantaged individually owned accounts that let individuals save pre-tax dollars for future qualified medical expenses.

high deductible health plan (HDHP): If you enroll in an HDHP, you may pay a lower monthly premium but have a higher deductible (meaning individuals pay for more of their health-care items and services before the insurance plan pays).

home care aide: Home care aides assist with nonmedical needs that require no prescription. They provide companionship and are usually people who have obtained some training to provide assistance with activities of daily living (ADLs). They help care for physically or mentally ill, injured, disabled, or infirm individuals who are confined to their homes or living in residential care facilities. They may also provide daily care services to people with disabilities who work outside the home.

home health aide: Rather than doctors, nurses are typically the ones who visit homes to treat illnesses. Nurses will consult with the primary care doctor to set up a plan of care, which might include medication administration, intravenous therapy, pain control, and so on.

immediate annuities: Immediate annuities are purchased with a one-time contribution and provide income payments to the annuitant within one year of purchasing the contract.

immediate fixed annuity: Immediate fixed annuity contracts provide annuitants a fixed income stream based, in part, from the interest rate guarantee at the time of purchase.

impaired risk: An impaired risk is any health condition or related factor that is likely to reduce someone's longevity.

impaired risk rider: If you have a health condition or injury that is expected to shorten your life span, an impaired risk rider is a provision that will accelerate the income payments in an annuity.

indemnity payout: Per the contract, monthly payments of a fixed amount, regardless of incurred care costs, are paid out.

indexed annuity: Indexed annuity contracts have both fixed and variable features. Under these policies, interest credits are linked to an external index of investments, such as bonds or the S&P 500, and usually contain a minimum guaranteed interest rate.

individual retirement account (IRA): An IRA is a tax-advantaged account that individuals use to save and invest for retirement.

inflation protection or inflation rider: Inflation protection is generally designed to protect the value of the dollar benefit from being eroded over time. It is a feature in which the value of benefits increases by a predefined percentage at specific time periods to help policyholders make sure that the benefits they receive can keep up with general price levels.

insurance: Insurance is a contract, represented by a policy, in which an individual or entity receives from an insurance company financial protection or reimbursement against losses. The company pools clients' risks to make payments more affordable for the insured.

insurance claim: An insurance claim is a formal request by a policyholder to an insurance company for coverage or compensation for a covered loss or policy event.

interest rate: An interest rate is the amount a lender charges for the use of assets expressed as a percentage of the principal. The interest rate is typically noted on an annual basis, known as the annual percentage rate (APR). Very low interest rates can make it very difficult for insurers, retirees, and other risk-averse investors to achieve the returns they anticipate.

Internal Revenue Code (IRC): The IRC is the domestic portion of federal statutory tax law in the United States, and it is under Title 26 of the United States Code (USC). The IRC is the governing law of federal tax administration and collection.

investment advisor: An investment advisor is a person or firm that is engaged in the business of providing investment advice to others or issuing reports or analyses regarding securities for compensation. Investment advisers generally must register with the Securities and Exchange Commission (SEC) or state securities authorities.

lapse or lapsation rates: A lapse is the expectation that people will cancel their policies or die before payment of claims.

level term, or level-premium, policies: Level term policies provide coverage for a specified period ranging from ten to thirty years. Both the death benefit and premium are fixed.

lien method chronic illness riders: A lien is established against the death benefit. Future premiums or charges for the coverage are not affected, and the gross cash value continues to grow as if the lien did not exist. With this method, an individual is, in effect, taking a loan against a future death benefit payout and has to pay interest on that loan. Expense charges may be added to the lien.

life insurance: There are two basic types of life insurance: term insurance and cash value insurance. There are many types of life insurance that can carry riders. The Life Insurer's Buyer's Guide prepared by the National Association of insurance Commissioners offers definitions.

lifetime maximum dollar benefit: The lifetime maximum dollar benefit, or lifetime limits, refers to the maximum dollar amount that an insurance company agrees to pay for covered services per the policy contract agreement.

longevity: Longevity refers to how long someone can reasonably expect to live.

longevity risk: Longevity risk is the likelihood that someone will outlive their financial resources.

long-term care benefit rider (LTCBR): LTCBRs combines two riders. Rather than separate accelerated death benefit and extension of benefits riders, the LTCBR allows for a streamlined contract structure and consistent pricing between the benefit period options.

long-term care policies: Long-term care insurance policies are not standardized. Instead, insurers sell policies that provide a variety of benefits. Every insurer must define its terms, benefits, and exclusions in the policy. Insurers must also deliver an outline of coverage that helps explain these terms to a prospective buyer.

maximum daily benefit amount: The daily benefit amount (DBA) is the maximum amount a contract will pay per day for covered services.

morbidity: In insurance lingo, morbidity refers to having a disease or a symptom of a disease.

mortality: Mortality refers to the state of being mortal or destined to die.

National Association of Insurance Commissioners (NAIC): The NAIC strives to protect the public interest, promote competitive markets, and improve the state regulation of insurance.

Omnibus Reconciliation Act (OBRA): The Omnibus Reconciliation Act of 1993 disallowed the future granting of waivers from the Health and Human Services Department for the purpose of forming a RWJ Long-Term Care Partnership program.

Partnership for Long-Term Care, the RWJ Partnership program: The RWJ Partnership program is a joint federal-state policy initiative to promote the purchase of private long-term care insurance. Currently, these programs operate in four states: California, Connecticut, Indiana, and New York.

Partnership policies: In an attempt to incentivize more aging Americans to purchase a private LTC insurance policy, the Deficit Reduction Act (DRA) of 2005 included section 6021, which created the Qualified State Long-Term Care Partnership program.

patient care assistants or aides (PCA): PCAs work with patients under the direct supervision of health-care professionals, such as doctors or nurses. They help patients with tasks such as bathing, dressing, and eating. They also assist with taking patients' temperature, blood pressure, pulse, and respiration.

per diem limits*:* Annually, the Internal Revenue Service (IRS) announces the annual inflation-adjusted health savings account (HSA) contribution limits for the calendar year. It also outlines the minimum deductible as well as maximum out-of-pocket expenses for high deductible health plans (HDHPs).

preseentism: Preseentism is a term use to describe employees who seem to be physically present but mentally absent.

qualified annuity versus nonqualified annuity: The difference between a qualified or nonqualified annuity has nothing to do with the annuity product itself but rather the tax status of the funds used. Qualified annuities are purchased with pre-tax dollars. Nonqualified plans use post-tax dollars to fund them.

rated age: Rated age is something like a biological age—that is, it is an individual's age based on their actual physical condition.

rate-increased premium payments: Traditional long-term care policy premiums have incurred adjustments to premiums.

reimbursement: Once approved for benefits, an individual receives a benefit equal to the total cost of qualified services, up to the policy's predetermined maximum.

reinstatement provision: A reinstatement provision is a clause found in an insurance policy that grants the policyholder a limited period of time to reinstate their policy after it has lapsed.

residential care home: The level of care in residential care homes is generally considered relatively personal since one caregiver is usually assigned to three to four senior residents.

retirement earnings test: If an individual claims social security benefits before reaching full retirement age (FRA), continues to work, and earns above a certain threshold, they are subject to the retirement earnings test.[93]

return of premium (ROP): ROP is a type of benefit or rider that provides, under specified stated conditions, for the return of the premiums paid for coverage.

riders: A rider is supplemental to an insurance policy. It amends the policy to include optional terms or conditions. Sometimes these add-ons are built into the policy, and other times they are available at an additional cost.

Section 125 plan: Section 125 is the section of the IRS code that enables and allows employees to take taxable benefits, such as a cash salary, and convert them into nontaxable benefits. These benefit premiums may be deducted from an employee's paycheck before taxes are paid.

Shopper's Guide: The National Association of Insurance Commissioners (NAIC) wrote the Shopper's Guide to help consumers understand long-term care and the insurance options that can help pay for long-term care services. This, or a guide developed or approved by a state commissioner, must be provided to all prospective applicants of a long-term care insurance policy or certificate.

short-term care (STC): STC is sometimes referred to as recovery care and is generally purchased by older individuals, ages fifty to eighty-nine, to cover gaps in Medicare coverage or as an alternative to long-term care protection.

single premium immediate annuity (SPIA): A SPIA may also be called an income annuity, or simply an immediate annuity. When you purchase a SPIA, you trade a large, lump-sum premium payment up front for extended, periodic payouts from an insurance company or a similar institution.

tax-qualified policy: Individuals may be eligible for a tax deduction of a policy's premiums and benefits. Form 1099-LTC states that "amounts paid under a qualified long-term care insurance contract are excluded from your income."

term insurance: Unlike permanent insurance policies that are designed to insure the policyholder for a lifetime, term policies have no value other than the guaranteed death benefit and feature no savings component. Once the term expires, the policyholder may have the option to renew for another term. Another option may be to convert the policy to permanent coverage, but there may be limitations as to which policy is offered for conversion.

terminal illness rider: A terminal illness rider is an accelerated benefit rider that permits a policyholder to access a portion of the funds provided in the policy before death. Terminal illnesses have no known cure, or have progressed to a point where one can no longer be cured and death is expected within months rather than years.

third-party notification or unintentional lapse protection: A person who is not the insured is contacted after the premium is late by a specified number of days.

traditional long-term care insurance (TLTC): TLTC may also be referred to as standalone LTC. Some advisors refer to it as pure protection since, unlike some other insurance options where policies combine different coverages, TLTC focuses solely on offsetting expenses for an extended or long-term care need.

transitional care assistance (TCA) benefit: A TCA benefit helps clients transition from informal to formal care.

underwriting: Underwriting is the process through which a company or institution takes on financial risk for a fee. Underwriters look for risks that could shorten life span or health risks that could cause claims early in the premium-paying years.

underwriting classes: Underwriting classes separate people into risk groups. The risk group or classification, also known as a risk class, is used to determine the premium of an insurance policy.

universal life insurance: Universal life insurance is a kind of flexible policy that lets you vary your premium payments and adjust the face amount of your coverage. Increases may require proof that you qualify for the new death benefit.

variable annuity: A variable annuity contract allows the policy owner to allocate contributions into various subaccounts of a separate account based on the risk appetite of the annuitant. Policyholders assume the investment risk with variable annuities.

variable life insurance: Variable life insurance is a kind of insurance where the death benefits and cash values depend on the investment performance of one or more separate accounts, which may be invested in mutual funds or other investments permitted under the policy. The insurer provides a prospectus for this type of policy.

waiver of premium clause or rider: The waiver of premium clause waives premium payments if the policyholder becomes critically ill, seriously injured, or disabled. Other stipulations may apply, such as meeting specific health and age requirements.

whole life insurance: Whole life insurance covers an individual for their lifetime as long as policy premiums are paid.

worksite long-term care: Employers of all types and sizes may offer a long-term care insurance benefit program. The worksite market has expanded to include hybrid/combo/linked sales as well as individual policies and group certificates sold with discounts and/or underwriting concessions to qualifying groups of people based on common employment.

ENDNOTES

1   Betty Meredith, CFA®, CFP®, CRC® 847-686-0440 x102 http://www.retirement-speakers-bureau.com.

2   "Longevity and Retirement: An Expert on Aging Explains How Retirement Is Being Redefined," Fidelity Viewpoints, Fidelity, February, 3, 2021, https://www.fidelity.com/viewpoints/retirement/longevity.

3   "Silent Generation," Wikipedia, https://en.wikipedia.org/wiki/Silent_Generation#:~:text=The%20Silent%20Generation%20is%20the,United%20States%20as%20of%202019.

4   Dana Anspach, reviewed by Marguerita Cheng, "What Retirement Is and How to Get There," The Balance, updated August 29, 2021, https://www.thebalance.com/what-is-retirement-2388822

5   Liz Seegert, "New Data Updates the Economic Value of Family Caregiving," Covering Health (blog), Association of Health Care Journalists, November 15, 2019, https://healthjournalism.org/blog/2019/11/new-data-updates-the-economic-value-of-family-caregiving/.

6   Merrill Silverstein and Roseann Giarrusso, "Aging and Family Life: A Decade Review," accessed May 9, 2021, https://www.ncbi.nim.nih.gov/pmc/articles/PMC3427733.

7   National Institute on Aging, "Long-Distance Caregiving: Twenty Questions and Answers," accessed May 25, 2021, https://order.nia.nih.gov/sites/default/files/2017-07/L-D-Caregiving_508.pdf

8   Liz Seegert, "New Data Updates the Economic Value of Family Caregiving," https://healthjournalism.org/blog/2019/11/new-data-updates-the-economic-value-of-family-caregiving/.

[9]   Richard Eisenberg (contributor), "The Financial and Personal Toll of Family Caregiving," Forbes, March 12, 2018, https://www.forbes.com/sites/nextavenue/2018/03/12/the-financial-and-personal-toll-of-family-caregiving/?sh=46c30d9858b8.

[10] Embracingcarers.com "Embracing Carers US survey," 2017, accessed April 21, 2021, https://www.embracingcarers.com/content/dam/web/healthcare/corporate/embracingcarers/media/infographics/us/Embracing%20Carers%0US%20Survey%20Results%20KGaA_FINAL.pdf.

[11] "Caregiver Stress," Office on Women's Health, US Department of Health and Human Services, https://www.womenshealth.gov/a-z-topics/caregiver-stress.

[12] Richard W. Johnson, "What Is the Lifetime Risk of Needing and Receiving Long-term Services and Supports?" April 4, 2019, https://aspe.hhs.gov/basic-report/what-lifetime-risk-needing-and-receiving-Long-term-services-and-supports.

[13] The National Clearinghouse for Long-Term Care information website was developed by the US Department of Health and Human Services, accessed April 21, 2021, https://www.healthinaging.org/tools-and-tips/national-clearinghouse-Long-term   careinformation#:~:text=The%20National%20Clearinghouse%20for%20Long,term%20care%20(LTC)%20needs.

[14] Estimate based on a hypothetical couple retiring in 2020, sixty-five years old, with life expectancies that align with Society of Actuaries' RP-2014 Healthy Annuitant rates with Mortality Improvements Scale MP-2016. Actual assets needed may be more or less depending on actual health status, area of residence, and longevity. Estimate is net of taxes. The Fidelity Retiree Health Care Cost Estimate assumes individuals do not have employer-provided retiree health-care coverage but do qualify for the federal government's insurance program, Original Medicare. The calculation takes into account cost-sharing provisions (such as deductibles and coinsurance) associated with Medicare Part A and Part B (inpatient and outpatient medical insurance). It also considers Medicare Part D (prescription drug coverage) premiums and out-of-pocket costs, as well as certain services excluded by Original Medicare. The estimate does not include other health-related expenses, such as over-the-counter medications, most dental services, and long-term care.

[15] Ibid.

[16] "How to plan for Rising Health Care Costs," Fidelity Viewpoints, Fidelity, May 6, 2021, https://fidelity.com/viewpoints/personal-finance/

plan-for-rising-health-care-costs With respect to federal taxation only. Contributions, investment earnings, and distributions may or may not be subject to state taxation. Please consult with your tax advisor regarding your specific situation.

17 Susan Reinhard, Lynn Friss Feinberg, Ari Houser, Rita Choula, Molly Evans, "Valuing the Invaluable 2019 Update: Charting a Path Forward," Public Policy Institute," November 14, 2019, AARP, https://www. aarp.org/content/dam/aarp/ppi/2019/11/valuing-the-invaluable-2019-update-charting-a-path-forward.doi.10.26419-2Fppi.00082.001.pdf pg.1.

18 "Caregiver Statistics: Work and Caregiving," Family Caregiver Alliance, National Center on Caregiving, https://www.caregiver.org/caregiver-statistics-work-and-caregiving.

19 "Elder Financial Exploitation," National Adult Protective Services Association, https://www.napsa-now.org/get-informed/exploitation-resources/.

20 The Conversation Project National Survey, 2018, accessed May 10, 2021, https://theconversationproject.org/.

21 "10 Shocking Statistics About Elderly Falls," Senior Health and Wellness Blog, Shell Point Retirement Community, accessed September 27, 2020, https://www.shellpoint.org/blog/10-shocking-statistics-about-elderly-falls/.

22 Susan Reinhard, Lynn Friss Feinberg, Ari Houser, Rita Choula, Molly Evans, Public Policy Institute," November 14, 2019, AARP, https://www.aarp.org/content/dam/aarp/ppi/2019/11/valuing-the-invaluable-201 9-update-charting-a-path-forward.doi.10.26419-2Fppi.00082.001.pdf pg.1.

23 Ibid., 5

24 *May 20, 2015 (Shared Services) | U.S. Department of Commerce* https:// www.commerce.gov/hr/practitioners/labor-management/forum/may-20-2015-meeting "Caregiving in the U.S. 2020," The National Alliance for Caregiving, accessed May 15, 2021, https://www.caregiving.org/caregiving-in-the-us-2020/.

25 "Wired for Care: The New Face of Caregiving in America," Cambia Health Solutions, accessed May 5, 2021, https://www.cambiahealth.com/newsroom/resources/wired-care-new-face-caregiving-america-0

26 Genworth, Cost of Care by State, Cost of Care Report, Home / Aging & You / Aging & Your Finances / Cost of Care
https://www.genworth.com/aging-and-you/finances/cost-of-care.html
https://www.lfg.com/public/individual/exploreinsuranceannuities/longtermcareplanning/thecosticc
https://www.oneamerica.com/caresolutionscalculator/index.html

27 "Drivers of the Cost of Care," Genworth, accessed May 10, 2021, https://www.genworth.com/aging-and-you/finances/cost-of-care/cost-of-care-trends-and-insights.html

28 National Academy of Elder Care Attorneys, https://www.naela.org/findlawyer.

29 "How to Plan for Rising Health Care Costs," Fidelity Viewpoints, May 6, 2021, https://www.fidelity.com/viewpoints/personal-finance/plan-for-rising-health-care-costs.
With respect to federal taxation only. Contributions, investment earnings, and distributions may or may not be subject to state taxation. Please consult with your tax advisor regarding your specific situation.

30 Social Security Administration, accessed June 22, 2020, http://www.ssa.gov. Worker benefits and spousal benefits are based on full retirement age (FRA)—sixty-six years (birth years 1943 to 1954), sixty-six years and two months to sixty-six years and ten months (1955 to 1959), and sixty-seven years (1960 and later).

31 Social Security Quick Calculator, Social Security Online, www.ssa.gov/OACT/quickcalc

32 "Compare Savings Options," Saving for College, https://www.savingforcollege.com/compare_savings_options/?assigned_to%5B%5D=0&assigned_to%5B%5D=5&hiddenField=vehicles&mode=Submit.

33 Courtesy of Dan Mangus, dan.mangus@smsteam.net, 800-689-2800, https://www.smsteam.net

34 https://www.medicare.gov/coverage/long-term-care

35 "What's Medicare Supplement Insurance (MediGap)?" Medicare.Gov, https://www.medicare.gov/supplements-other-insurance/whats-medicare-supplement-insurance-medigap

36 https://www.insure.com/health-insurance/long-term-care-medicare-advantage

37 Aleesha Lockett, "How Is Medicare Funded?" Healthline, May 28, 2020. https://www.healthline.com/health/medicare/how-is-medicare-funded

38 https://www.medicaid.gov/medicaid/financialmanagement/index.html#:~:text=The%20Medicaid%20program%20is%20jointly,Medical%20Assistance%20Percentage%20(FMAP).

39 https://www.medicaid.gov/coverage/long-term-care

40 Courtesy of Dan Mangus, dan.mangus@smsteam.net, 800-689-2800, https://www.smsteam.net

41 Kim Parker and Eileen Patten, "The Sandwich Generation: Rising Financial Burdens for Middle-Aged Americans," The Pew Research Center, January 30, 2013, https://www.pewresearch.org/social-trends/2013/01/30/the-sandwich-generation/

42 PMC, US National Library of Medicine National Institutes of Health, Published online 2017 Nov 11. doi: 10.1093/geroni/igx025 accessed 6/22/2020 https://www.ncbi.nlm.nih.gov/pmc/articles/PMC5954612/

43 Richard Fry, "Millennials Overtake Baby Boomers as America's Largest Generation," Pew Research Center, 04/28/2020, https://www.pewresearch.org/fact-tank/2020/04/28/millennials-overtake-baby-boomers-as-americas-largest-generation/-:~:text=Millennials overtake Baby Boomers as America's largest generation&text=Millennials have surpassed Baby Boomers,from the U.S. Census Bureau.

44 Chuck Rainville, Laura Skufca, and Laura Mehegan. *Family Caregiving and Out-of-Pocket Costs: 2016 Report*, Washington, DC: AARP Research, November 2016. https://doi.org/10.26419/res.00138.001.

45 Retirement Benefits Estimator, Social Security Administration, https://www.ssa.gov/benefits/retirement/estimator.html.

46 NSSA, National Social Security Advisor, https://www.nationalsocialsecurityassociation.com or NARSSA, the National Association of Registered Social Security Analysts, https://www.narssa.org

47 Retirement and Survivors Benefits: Life Expectancy Calculator, Social Security Administration, https://www.ssa.gov/oact/population/longevity.html.

48 Kim Parker, Rich Morin, and Juliana Menasce Horowitz, "Looking to the Future, Public Sees an America in Decline on Many Fronts," U.S. Department of Health and Human Services, accessed October 16, 2020, https://longtermcare.acl.gov/the-basics/how-much-care-will-you-need.html

49 The Four Pillars of the New Retire*ment*, Edward Jones (website), accessed October 3, 2020, https://app.getresponse.com/click.html?x=a62b&lc=B3d-jyv&mc=Ic&s=UK8VfB&u=BRtag&z=EM5kzVD&.

50 "Half of Retirees Say They Wish They'd Budgeted More for This, " Fox Business, September 26, 2020, https://app.getresponse.com/click.html?x=a62b&lc=B3djGb&mc=Ic&s=UK8VfB&u=BRtag&z=E91VCHy&

51 "Generational Attitudes and Behaviour," The Nordic Page, accessed October 3, 2020, https://www.tnp.no/norway/global/2859-generational-attitudes-and-behaviour#:~:text=A%20generation%20can%20be%20considered,their%20thinking%20and%20behavior%20today.&text=

Generation%20Y%20are%20the%20children,born%20between%20
1980%20and%201999

52 Kristen Bialik and Richard Fry, "Millennial Life: How Young Adulthood
    Today Compares with Prior Generations," Pew Research Center, January
    30,   2019,   https://www.pewresearch.org/social-trends/2019/02/14/
    millennial-life-how-young-adulthood-today-compares-with-prior-
    generations-2/

53 "Retirement Benefits," Social Security Administration, accessed, October
    7, 2020. https://www.ssa.gov/benefits/retirement/planner/1943.html

54 My Social Security account page, Social Security Administration, accessed
    October 7, 2020, https://www.ssa.gov/myaccount/.

55 "States, Counties, and Statistically Equivalent Entities," Google, Chapter 4,
    accessed 10/08/2020 https://www.google.com/search?q=number+of+coun-
    ties+in+the+us&oq=number+of+counties+in+the+US&aqs=chrome.0.0i45
    7j0j0i22i30l3.22668j0j15&sourceid=chrome&ie=UTF-8

56 https://www.genworth.com/aging-and-you/finances/cost-of-care.html
    https://www.lfg.com/public/individual/exploreinsuranceannuities/
    longtermcareplanning/thecosticc
    https://www.oneamerica.com/caresolutionscalculator/index.html

57 IRS Publication 502, which contains a list of allowable expenses and IRS
    publication 969, accessed November 8, 2020, http://IRS.gov

58 IRS Publication 969, Health Savings Accounts and Other Tax-Favored
    Health Plans, Internal Revenue Service, accessed November 8, 2020,
    https://www.irs.gov/publications/p969. Telehealth and other remote care
    coverage with plan years beginning before 2022 is disregarded for deter-
    mining who is an eligible individual. (CARES Act, P. L. 116-136, March
    27, 2020).

59 Tina Orem, How FICA Tax and Tax Withholding Works in 2021,
    NerdWallet,   May   4,2021,   https://www.nerdwallet.com/article/taxes/
    fica-tax-withholding

60 Kimberly Lankford, "Using a Health Savings Account to Pay Long-Term-
    Care Premiums," Kiplinger, accessed November 8, 2020, https://www.
    kiplinger.com/article/insurance/t027-c001-s003-using-a-hsa-to-pay-long-
    term-care-premiums.html

61 Revenue Procedure 2020-32, Internal Revenue Service, accessed November
    15, 2020, http://irs.gov/pub/irs-drop/rp-20-32.pdf. The IRS confirms HSA
    contribution limits effective for each calendar year. The IRS confirms HSA
    contribution limits effective for 2021, along with minimum deductible and
    maximum out-of-pocket expenses for the HDHPs with which HSAs are

paired. Additional resource- Stephen Miller, "IRS Announces 2021 Limits for HSAs and High-Deductible Health Plans," SHRM, May 21, 2020, https://www.shrm.org/resourcesandtools/hr-topics/benefits/pages/irs-2021-hsa-contribution-limits.aspx.

62 There are exceptions with regard to eligibility for opening individual an HSA account. Someone who is already covered by another health plan or is at least sixty-five years old and enrolled in Medicare, or is claimed as a dependent on someone else's tax return, cannot open an HSA.

63 HSA Search (website), accessed November 21, 2020, http://www.hsa-search.com.

64 Tina Orem, How FICA Tax and Tax Withholding Works in 2021, NerdWallet, May 4, 2021, https://www.nerdwallet.com/article/taxes/fica-tax-withholding

65 NAIFA's Limited and Extended Care Planning Center, NAIFA, accessed November 21, 2020, lecp.naifa.org

66 Larry Rubin, FSA, CERA, MAAA: PricewaterhouseCoopers, Partner Kevin Crowe, CPA: PricewaterhouseCoopers, Partner Adam Fisher: PricewaterhouseCoopers Omar Ghaznawi: PricewaterhouseCoopers Richard McCoach: PricewaterhouseCoopers Rachel Narva, ASA: PricewaterhouseCoopers David Schaulewicz: PricewaterhouseCoopers Tom Sullivan Toby White, FSA, CFA, Ph.D.,, "An Overview of the U.S. LTC Insurance Market (Past and Present): The Economic Need for LTC Insurance, the History of LTC Regulation & Taxation and the Development of LTC Product Design Features," Society of Actuaries, accessed 11/22/2020

67 Blog / Insurance Claim Denied / A Brief History of Long-term care Insurance, (August 25,2017), accessed 11/22/2020, https://turbaklaw.com/a-brief-history-of-Long-term-care-insurance/

68 Larry Rubin, FSA, CERA, MAAA, Partner Kevin Crowe, CPA, Partner Adam Fisher, Omar Ghaznawi, Richard McCoach, Rachel Narva, ASA, David Schaulewicz, Tom Sullivan, Toby White, FSA, CFA, Ph.D.: Drake University, Associate Professor of Actuarial Science, "An Overview of the U.S. LTC Insurance Market (Past and Present): The Economic Need for LTC Insurance, the History of LTC Regulation & Taxation and the Development of LTC Product Design Features," accessed 7/22/2020 https://www.soa.org/globalassets/assets/files/resources/essays-monographs/managing-impact-ltc/mono-2014-ltc-manage-narva.pdf

69 "A Brief History of Long-term care Insurance," Turbak Law Office, P.C., August 25, 2017, https://turbaklaw.com/a-brief-history-of-Long-term-care-insurance/.

70 "The Deficit Reduction Act: Important Facts for State & Local Government Officials," CMS. gov, accessed July 22, 2020, https://www.cms.gov/Regulations-and-Guidance/Legislation/DeficitReductionAct/Downloads/Guide.pdf

71 "Long-term Care Partnership Expansion: A New Opportunity for States" (Issue Brief), May 2007, https://www.chcs.org/media/Long-term_Care_Partnership_Expansion.pdf.

72 "The Many Faces of Caregivers: A Close-Up Look at Caregiving and Its Impacts," Transamerica Center for Retirement Studies, Transamerica Institute, accessed November 22, 2020, https://www.transamericacenter.org/retirement-research/caregiver-research.

73 Amy Bell, reviewed by Thomas J. Catalano, "How Cash Value Builds in a Life Insurance Policy," Investopedia, updated January 2, 2021, https://www.investopedia.com/articles/personal-finance/082114/how-cash-value-builds-life-insurance-policy.asp

74 "Understanding the Different Types of Annuities," insuranceandestates.com, updated June 1, 2019, https://www.insuranceandestates.com/annuity/.

75 Bloomberg Tax, IRC/Subtitle A/Chapter1/Subchapter B/Part II/§ 72 https://irc.bloombergtax.com/public/uscode/doc/irc/section_72

76 Elaine Silvestrini, financially reviewed by Rubina Hossain, CFP®, "Qualified vs. Non-Qualified Annuities," Annuity.org, accessed August 15, 2020, https://www.annuity.org/annuities/taxation/qualified-vs-nonqualified/.

77 You may not qualify for critical or chronic illness accelerated death benefits if your health is rated too far below a certain underwriting risk classification or if you have a specific health condition that requires an extra premium charge known as a "medical flat extra." Terminal illness coverage has the same criteria as the life insurance policy issued. If you qualify for life insurance coverage, then the terminal illness accelerated death benefit endorsement will be issued with the policy.

78 content.naic.org, attachment B, accessed January 3, 2021, https://content.naic.org/sites/default/files/national_meeting/Health%20Insurance%20Committee%20Fall%20National%20Mtg%20Minutes.pdf.

79 "General Attitudes and Behaviour," The Nordic Page, accessed November 3, 2020, https://www.tnp.no/norway/global/2859-generational-attitudes-and-behaviour#:~:text=A%20generation%20can%20be%20considered,their%20thinking%20and%20behavior%20today.&text=

Generation%20Y%20are%20the%20children,born%20between%20 1980%20and%201999.

80 Omri Wallach, *Charting the Growing Generational Wealth Gap*, December 2, 2020, www.visualcapilalist.com.

81 "A New Financial Reality," PEW, September 18, 2014, https://www. pewtrusts.org/en/research-and-analysis/reports/2014/09/a-new-financial-reality.

82 American Council of Life Insurers. Long-term care and Disability Income. p.81 https://www.acli.com/-/media/ACLI/Files/Fact-Books-Public/9FB18Chapter9DILTC.ashx?la=en

83 Form 1099, IRS, https://www.irs.gov/forms-pubs/about-form-1099-ltc. The True Cost of Forgotten 401(k) Accounts, June 2, 2021, accessed February 7, 2021 https://www.hicapitalize.com>resources>the-true-cost-of-forgotten-401ks/

84 Courtesy of Joe Dowdall, CFP®, RICP®, MBA, CRPC® Financial Advisor 214-578-5884 Joe@worthassetmgmt.com

85 Sara Rabi, "401(k) or IRA? That Is the Question," November 5, 2020, http://www.wealthmanagement.com.

86 "Should You Exchange Your Life Insurance Policy," FINRA.org, accessed December 22, 2020, https://www.finra.org/investors/alerts/should-you-exchange-your-life-insurance-policy

87 "Exchange Rules," Google. https://www.google.com/search?q=1035+-exchange+rules&oq=1035+exchang&aqs=chrome.2.35i39j69i-57j0l6.9924j0j15&sourceid=chrome&ie=UTF-8

88 www.lecp.naifa.org or www.naifa.org under Centers tab

89 Certification For Long-term care. Google. https://www.ltc-cltc.com

90 *A Shopper's Guide to Long-term care Insurance*, National Association of Insurance Commissioners (NAIC), accessed February 8, 2021, https:// www.naic.org/documents/prod_serv_consumer_ltc_lp.pdf

91 Courtesy LTCI Partners, LLC http://www.ltcipartners.com Steve Cain, steve.cain@ltcipartners.com (608) 283-6600

92 https://www.cdc.gov/phlp/publications/topic/hipaa.html

93 https://www.ssa.gov/policy/docs/program-explainers/retirement-earnings-test.html; https://www.aarp.org/retirement/planning-for-retirement/info-2018/going-back-to-work-ss.html